SIMPLE STRUCTURED TRAINING
How The Mind Builds The Body

ISBN: 978-0-9907776-0-1

Published by TypinInc, Warren, Michigan

DEDICATION

This book is dedicated to the neighborhood friends and families who taught me how to play in those days when that's all I had to do was play; Dave, Tim, Bry, Jeff, Doug, Wes, Bob and the rest of the Beierman Block.

To all the coaches, parents, cheerleaders and supporters on the sidelines who watched while the mud and blood stuck to our tired smiles; because being a part of something was always better than being apart.

To the Bad Dudes of Sigma Alpha Epsilon Delta Chapter, '75-79; who went undefeated in every sport, nearly every year we were at Western. We had some fun, and learned some, too.

To the Center Line 7; Dan G, Dan T, John, Carl, Elliot, Brad & Aaron, whom were my test rats for this wicked experiment as I developed and refined these methods.

To my sons; Thomas, Zachary & Spencer, who always remind me what energy and spirit and sport do to keep the soul young; and finally, to my wife Deborah for the love, support and space a writer needs to write. This was definitely a marathon experience.

SIMPLE STRUCTURED TRAINING -
Table of Contents

A sound mind in a sound body. – Aristotle - 345 B.C.

SHOW SIMPLICITY, HOLD FAST TO HONESTY –LAO TZU

Thirty spokes surround the hub:

In their nothingness consists the carriage's effectiveness.

One hollows the clay and shapes it into pots:

In its nothingness consists the pot's effectiveness.

One cuts out doors and windows to make the chamber:

In their nothingness consists the chamber's effectiveness.

Therefore, what exists serves for possession

What does not exist serves for effectiveness.

What is half shall become whole

What is crooked shall become straight

What is empty shall become full.

What is old shall become new.

Whosoever has little shall receive

Whosoever has much, from him shall be taken away.

Whosoever knows others is clever

Whosoever knows himself is wise.

Whosoever conquers others has force.

Whosoever conquers himself is strong.

Whosoever asserts himself has will power.

Whosoever is self-sufficient is rich.

Whosoever does not lose his place has duration.

Whosoever does not perish in death lives.

A stanza of this poem accompanies each chapter in this book, aligning thoughts and requesting an honest assessment of where your present condition is, in order for you to get to where you desire.

SIMPLE STRUCTURED

TRAINING

Introduction

What you hold in your hands is a guidebook to better athletic performance and intelligent attention toward life. Simple Structured Training contains the training necessary for all sports at all levels. This book benefits athletes with techniques for strength, stability, flexibility and transformation. It teaches you to dwell on the weaknesses until they become strengths.

In a non-competitive vein, the everyday tasks of carrying groceries, picking up children or working in an environment with repetitive movements can be enhanced by paying attention to what your life does to your body on a daily basis, and how Simple Structured Training can turn obstructions into pathways. As long as your life contains gravity, you can benefit from Simple Structured Training. Strength comes from the self-assurance of making the "eventful" the "every day." Repeatedly proving your own capabilities ingrains success, until even failing is welcomed because it shows where work needs attention. Training means making practice harder than a game can ever be, so the game becomes an event played at its highest level, always, and the body flies as it should, on autopilot.

Just as the concert pianist practices so as to not make a mistake the day of the concert, the athlete practices, and on game day, plays flawlessly. Practice and training come in many forms, from visualization to single maximum effort. But just like the artist, the athlete must let creativity and intuition win from time to time so "happy accidents" will manifest into higher insights of what the body and its performance can achieve. By occasionally deviating from the normal methods of sets and repetitions, the athlete learns about his body through open-mindedness, as the "feel" of certain movements register in the brain as well as the body.

EVERYBODY HAS A SPORT

Every person has a sport, be it working with weights or walking, tennis or triathlon. By taking a subjective look at yourself, applying the stepping stones of training from the core of what you have to start with, to higher and higher goals of what you can feasibly obtain, every person can improve their performance, lifestyle and health by paying attention to what they are doing to their bodies at work and at play.

Small adjustments in focus can brighten the big picture of what proper training can do for you. With the growing number of athletes involved in organized or recreational sports, and the variety of activities and equipment available to them, the need for balance, definitive plans and guidelines for achievement are absolutely necessary for safe, healthy progress.

Many aspects contribute to superior performance, from breathing to body mechanics, from how much and what goes into your body, to what comes out from it in terms of energy expenditure. Intelligently reviewing these aspects on a periodic basis, adjusting nutrition, exercise and rest in proportion to available time, and carrying through with plans, goals and scheduled routines to the end, will garner higher results, greater rewards, safer techniques, a wider knowledge base and stronger approaches toward every sport, every season.

YOU ARE A COMPETITOR

Competing with yourself is the ultimate struggle. We do it daily on many levels. Attending your workouts makes attending meetings, appointments, presentations and anything else easier, because confident, positive action started you off fresh, first thing in the morning.

You have to prove to yourself that you are the one in control of your day, your diet, your direction, your health. Take the time to take care of yourself, first thing in the morning. Start your day with silence, darkness, calm introspection, a good breakfast, a powerful thought, an attitude of being in control rather than frantically setting out in opposition to all the things vying for your time and attention. By taking charge from the outset, by writing dreams, praying, meditating, stretching, lightly exercising, going inward before going outward, turning everything off instead of on, you will accomplish all the to-do's on your list with little effort. Life will yank on you from every handle you give it. But if you choose to pull your own weight, you'll choose which direction you'll go, what you'll do first, and what you'll discard.

As long as we eat, move and breathe, we must exercise. And we must do it before injuries occur, on the front end, to ensure maximum health, happiness and productive contribution. If you're here to stay, than so too should your workouts or some type of physical activity, every day. The sooner you rest this in your mind, that exercise is just as essential to life as sleeping and eating, the faster you can find an activity which both meets your activity level and style.

Walking is exercise. Biking is exercise. Even gardening is exercise with its reaching and pulling, lifting and moving. If it fits your lifestyle and you enjoy it, stop begrudging it as "work" and respect the benefits available in everyday things. But learn how to do them safely, and to get the most from them, so they benefit your body as well as your mind.

IT BEGINS AND ENDS WITH "YOU"

Simple Structured Training starts with the equipment necessary for every sport and activity that you currently have and always will have - *your body*. People complain that they can't get to a gym, don't have the equipment, or can't work out alone because they need a spotter or partner to assist them, motivate them, support them.

Simple Structured Training teaches you how to use your bodyweight as its own resistance when you begin a strength training program. Once you learn how to add repetitions and sets to a foundation based on good form, you learn how to build on a program that disciplines your body in every area, alleviating weaknesses and building strength upon strength for better athletic performance, better health, longevity and lifelong activity.

**Simple Structured Training** works on the weaknesses hidden or ignored which hold you back from superior performance. It increases vertical and horizontal leap distances, directional mobility, and explosive power. Yet, it is simply a collection of exercises known by man for as long as they'd had a name for them. You must think of how you're currently training, why you are training, and if that training is effective enough to help you improve in your sport and your life.

**Simple Structured Training** asks you why and how you train in the first place. When you learn how your body works toward your respective activity, you begin to look at the movements you rehearse in practice so that performance becomes automatic on the field and reaction comes first rather than reflexion. This deep-seated mental acuity is key to making even the most simple work, play.

**Simple Structured Training** are a core group of exercises that everyone at every level should do. Balance, coordination, flexibility, strength, speed, agility, ability to recover, mental sharpness and physiological training are crucial at every age. As you train the body, you train the mind. You begin generally, learn, grow, feed-back, get more specific, and refine goals to continually monitor your plan until you get to a level of maintenance that fits both your time and physical demands.

What typically happens is that an athlete begins to favor the training he or she is stronger at, that which comes easier. Some would rather run than stretch, without realizing stretching would allow faster and longer runs. Some choose to strength train rather than run, not realizing the benefits of oxygen uptake on muscular endurance. The athlete that gets by on talent and genetics alone survives for a while with intermittent peak performances spotted by occasional injuries. The well-rounded athlete, who focuses on training weaknesses to strengths, while strengthening natural abilities, usually enjoys the longest career by constantly learning and achieving and often passing on this wealth of knowledge by example to others.

When you're tuned in to exactly how your muscles feel, you're doing it for you. If you're going too fast and not concentrating on the movement, you're doing it for a coach or condition, to just "get it done". Once you find yourself making it harder on purpose, pushing for extra reps, tuning in to how your body performs instead of taking motion for granted, you'll know you're hitting the upper levels of training. Going further, doing extra, paying attention and letting go reward the creative soul many times over. This "feel" is the basis of ***Simple Structured Training.***

INTENSITY

The understanding you'll need to be a better athlete is to simply feel what your body is telling you and respond to it with more or less intensity. Is your heart beating too fast as you exercise? Learn where your optimum heart rate should be for a given, desired outcome, then meet it, surpass it, or slow down. Do your joints ache? Pay attention to form, stance, angle, leverage and body position and back off on the weight. Is your bodyfat too high? Lower your intensity around food, and definitely skip the extra repetitions! There are no great secrets left to this training game. The major "bodybuilding," "shaping," "renewing," and "longevity" magazines have the same articles with the same exercises they had 50 years ago. They call it something else, wrap a concept around it, design new equipment and put a fresh-faced model next to it, but it's still Jack and Jill doing six basic movements.

People who get on a treadmill for forty minutes, four days in a week, after being physically dormant for 4 years, not only begin in an unbalanced state, but are bound to get more mechanically out of balance without flexibility training or working toward their maximum heart rate. Throw in some weight training with too little or too much resistance or incorrect execution, and you often have an injured athlete instead of a strong participant. With this, the frustration factor goes up, interest goes down and apathy returns because "you're hurt."

Many people work at jobs requiring them to bend, lift, lean, hunch, squat, or sit for hours on end. Some drive or travel daily, thousands of miles per year. Ergonomics in the office often only means a wrist rest near a computer keyboard, or an adjustable chair, while repetitive stresses are taking their toll on joints and organs. All areas of work, as well as play, can be enhanced by learning how to strengthen the posture and balance the symmetry.

STRENGTHEN THE POSTURE and BALANCE THE SYMMETRY

Notice how many people are hunched at the shoulders, slouched in their seats, uneven in their stride, top-heavy or bottom-heavy. The population is getting more and more out of balance at younger and younger ages.

How can a parent tell his child to stand up straight when his own shoulders are hunched or has a back in posterior tilt because of an oversized potbelly? Where are children supposed to learn to exercise daily when their gym teachers are 60, 70, 80 pounds overweight? How do you bring balance to lives filled with infrequent, non nutritious meals and sedentary excuses for play? You start by drawing a clear example, by leading rather than preaching.

Many people striving for fitness end up hindering their progress by a lack of balance. They should strive to balance their body symmetrically and increase their strength proportionately, in addition to enhancing lung capacity and endurance.

If your sport of choice requires club-speed, bat-speed, racquet speed or arm speed of any kind, than the surrounding muscles must be worked equally. Determine the speed and area of stride required for your sport. Running long, straight distances tax the body and its energy differently than short bursts of lateral or multidirectional movements. Mimicry of movement, such as weighted swings, are often detrimental to technique when overdone. All sports, played and participated in by all types and levels of athletes, gain unmatched athleticism when symmetry, strength and speed are garnered and gained through a balanced approach.

There are many people working to be fit, improve cardiovascular shape with marathon aspirations, become better defined or lighter and leaner, but the initial attention should go toward strengthening the posture and balancing the symmetry. Posture is the vertical alignment of your carriage. The structural integrity of your skeletal system is enhanced through

Pilates, chiropractic adjustment and strength training. They align the framework your flesh rests upon.

Symmetry is the top to bottom and left to right proportions. This is enhanced by yoga, massage and strength training. Pilates and chiropractic work the bones, while massage and yoga work the muscles. Strength training works both the bones and the muscles.

CONSISTENCY EQUALS RESULTS

If you make your workouts, cardio sessions and meal preparations with attentive frequency, you'll gain consistent results in strength, shape and health. You will never make consistent gains with inconsistent effort.

If your schedule requires fast, easy meals, take the effort to have on hand the best types of foods, prepared with the greatest benefit for nutritional input, so that you're adding to your health and energy rather than taking away from it. By choosing exercises that strengthen your weaknesses rather than always working "favorites," you alleviate the weak links that sooner than later materialize as injuries. By consistently using proper form on every plane, your shape will have more depth and therefore more appeal from every angle, in addition to functionality.

You must make a plan and work that plan, with enough common sense to know when to back off and when to add intensity. It does no good to show up and lazily go through the motions. If all you have to offer is 20 minutes of concentration, put what you've got into it and go home. Attend to the details. Exercise with attention to equal intention and leave when it falters.

The body responds to consistent effort. Train it often, as scheduled, and gains will result. Feed it in adequate amounts with rich, varied, whole foods and it responds with energy, alertness, slimness, longevity and a healthy immune response. Or, as too many are currently choosing, feed it with fat-laden, processed foods, poisonous tobacco, alcohol, soft drinks and empty calories and it responds as toxicity incarnate, with disease and debility.

If you train to become a better musician, you consistently work harder at practice and become a better player. An artist must create art by consistently practicing technique. An athlete must consistently prepare their body to the best of its capacity for performance, to become better athletes. That training never goes away. Just like music lessons, or artistic training, the daily ritual of practice lifts the play to uninhibited, unrestricted performance. Your body speaks a language and sometimes it shouts when it hurts and sometimes it whimpers when it's beaten, but it always responds to the stress put on it by accommodating and preparing for the next time that load is put in front of it. Consistency equals preparedness.

WHAT DO YOU WANT?

The first step with ***Simple Structured Training*** is to Think. You should be conscientious of what your body is going through on a daily basis.

- What do you want?
- How soon do you want it?
- How much are you ready to sacrifice to get it?
- How much time are you willing to invest in getting in shape?
- What equipment and facilities do you have to work with?
- What are you willing to learn?
- What are your ultimate goals?

It's no different than anything else in life. No one has anything new to offer. These revolutionary products on infomercials are simply new ways of taking your money with century old techniques of achieving your goal, like walking! Some books are full of cute phrases and new tags for old exercises, sit-ups are "Abdominal Abolishers."

So many books and videos are started with promises like, " In just 3 weeks…10 minutes…2 months, etc." What comes next? What happens after the 12-week workout – that wasn't suited to your body style in the first place – is over, and you're far short of the promised results? Do you know anything more about your body? Or did you just follow painted footsteps around on the gym floor for 3 months? If you're here to stay, than so too should your workouts and some type of physical activity, every day.

POETRY IN MOTION

The flexibility, the balance, the strength, the dexterity, the resilience, the blind bravery of a child is everyone's right. By ignoring your body through inactivity, by forgetting to play, you're really killing yourself. All the things keeping you from exercise or play don't compare to the benefits found with fitness. Every single aspect of your life, for all of your life, is positively affected when you put some thought and work into exercise and fitness.

As children, we experienced exhilaration and jubilation often enough to make it a natural thing in our growing lives. A drawing, a starred homework paper, a song, a cartwheel, a picture in the clouds, a hug, a fast bike ride home, a greeting from our dog, could each have been enough to trigger a feeling of that moment being more than ordinary life had to offer. Sometimes we noticed it, and sometimes it went by like the wind we ran through, but those magic moments were there for us to experience, and the feelings associated with them can be conjured for years to come in various situations.

Through our physical natures we transcend earth and achieve the spiritual. All athletes in all sports experience it at some time in their lives. The best athletes achieve it most often. There are many modes available for achieving this transcendence to the spiritual through the physical plane in competition. Dancers, artists, musicians, architects, writers and actors also experience this elevation by going deep within to bring out this magic, revelatory moment which inspires and awes others each time they're reviewed. This synchronistic execution of performance meeting preparation is the definition of "Poetry In Motion."

There's a reason these "things" are called "feelings." There's a reason victory and defeat bring equal tears of emotion. We are physical beings in three-dimensional space working on limited time. It is our privilege, blessing and duty to make the most of it. With **_Simple Structured Training_**, you can make the "eventful" the "everyday."

BE HONEST, FIND TRUTH

The poem by Lao Tzu, _Show Simplicity, Hold Fast To Honesty_, defines the essence of how Simple Structured Training should be approached, step-by-step, with clarity, vision and patience. Each age and culture have their own proponents of living the merits of an active life. From Socrates and Hippocrates to Tzu, Thoreau, Whitman, Lalane and Schwarzenegger, being in tune with our inner physicality accentuates the life lived on our exteriors, and resonates to those closest to us. As Einstein said, it is important to work only as much as it allows us to increase our leisure.

Life should be long. Give yourself enough time to find what works for you in keeping the physical aspects of your life working and intact. There is room for experiment. There is room for error. But there must be room for trial. I cannot help but stress how much an active life, especially one begun early, affects the way you look at everything from the simplest challenges, to the dreams and wishes you hold for your children.

Sporting events and our interest in them have grown tremendously. More schools have teams in more sports, with children specializing sooner in life. The Olympics add events annually. We have more food choices, more recreational outlets, more indulgences, yet more disease. Why not make your choices the ones that prove fruitful and beneficial to allow the longest, most abundant life possible across all aspects.

There is an Olympian in each one of us, whether we pursue that route or not, whether we'd even been to or seen an athletic event. As life courses through us, energy begets energy and the more we give, the more we get.

*"It is not enough that we do our best; sometimes
we have to do what is required."*
- Winston Churchill

1

<u>CORE</u>

"Thirty Spokes Surround The Hub:

In Their Nothingness

Consists The Carriage's

Effectiveness"

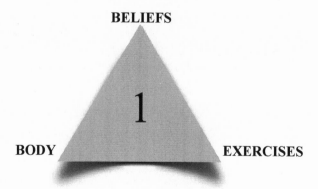

THE CORE IS THE FOUNDATION

In every sport, any exercise discipline, every form of learning, there is a core of knowledge that must be known before you can move on to the next level.

Our "spokes" are the arms, legs and head attached to the torso. Our appendages are extensions of the powers we emanate from the heart, mind and body centers. It's the spaces in between - the range of motion, movement, reach, stride, strength and grasp - that allow us to use our abilities to their highest benefit.

The "hub" is your core, your center of being. The important organs reside here. It is where you began and where you live or die. The heart, the stomach and the back are primary targets for injury and disease. Strength, stability, flexibility and explosiveness emanate from here. All forms of training have their basis and foundation in this core. When the core is strong, every other direction taken is strengthened proportionately. If one were to train just the outer spokes, the lopsided focus not only makes the center weaker, but each other subsequent direction more prone to accident or injury.

The "nothingness," therefore, can constitute rest, contemplation, visualization, feedback, non-doing, awareness and "nothingness." You push, you glide. This is the nothingness within the hub's "core." Utilize this "space" to grow mentally as well as physically.

The "effectiveness" of your training comes from working on your weaknesses, not your strengths. You want as few weaknesses as possible. You want to be balanced, fast, flexible, durable, strong and intuitive in every aspect. There will always be at least one dominant characteristic that stands out. Use that characteristic as inspiration to bring each other aspect up to par with that particular strength.

As energy emanates from the hub to the spokes, the spaces between compensate with proper responses. A well-rounded repertoire of training assures all aspects will act and react in correct proportion to the stress. The more well-trained the mind and body are, the more automatic the response. The "effectiveness" of the "carriage" is the result of efficient movement paired with automatic response emanating from a stable yet flexible base.

This Core Foundation is the initial building block that the rest of all training must be built upon. It is the stabilizing, beneath-the-surface, unseen aspect of physicality that transfers and distributes the opposing forces of gravity and inertia against the body into fluid movements which carry the body, and in return allow the body to utilize its own locomotion and force in its synchronistic dance of energy and movement.

The remaining ingredient is the spirit you bring to life to carry you toward your destination. Spirit is energy, it is attitude, it is intention, it is focus, it is discipline. It is knowing that somehow, some way, you will achieve what you've set out to receive. It is incorporating this foundational trine of *Belief, Body and Exercises* into any desire to rise above the average in competition or everyday better health.

C.O.R.E.

C *ONSISTENT* – You must participate, practice, and apply techniques regularly over a given amount of time.

O *RGANIZED* – With your plan in hand, your time is organized, and more gets done in less time, with measurable feedback.

R *EHEARSAL OF* – Practice until the movement becomes rote. To rehearse is to do over and over until both the mind and body respond automatically.

E *XERCISES* – Everything from the brain to the brawn must be conditioned. Exercise prepares the body to respond to certain stresses with force, flexibility, reaction and endurance.

THE CORE is what you begin the race with – your body.

THE CORE is the centerpiece, the power station from which energy originates.

THE CORE helps determine all speed and strength.

THE CORE is the most important element to train at all levels.

THE CORE is what you end the race with – your body.

THE CORE IS:

- *THE HEART* - This is where it all starts. If you're healthy here, everything will follow accordingly. If this suffers, so too will you until it's properly trained.
- *THE STOMACH* – The stabilizing force where your body turns from side to side, bends up and down, pushes, pulls and exerts force to the legs and arms.
- *THE LOWER BACK* – This is the opposing stabilizer to the stomach that must deal with momentum, inertia, counter-balance and forward movement, as well as supporting the body in its upright position.
- *THE HIPS* – Aid in turning the body, exerting force to change direction, absorbing shock, and stabilizing.

- *THE MUSCLES TYING THE FRONT TO THE BACK OF THE BODY* – This group – the serratus, intercostals and obliques – run through the center of the body and across the shoulders, tying the chest and stomach to the back and hips, creating a serape or cloak effect. These work together in forward, backward and lateral movements.

THE CORE BELIEFS

The Core Beliefs are where your goals, plans, visualizations, discipline, faith, feedback and truth come from. They're an intrinsic driving force that constantly tells you and you alone what you can or cannot do.

The Core Beliefs will either help you attain your goals, or keep you from them. If you have a lifelong wish to complete a marathon, do you believe you have the time to put in the necessary training to simply finish the race? Do you believe you can prepare yourself in the amount of time between now and the competition? Do you believe you are physically able to run the marathon? Do you believe you have the knowledge or access to it, to enable you to prepare properly and safely? Does your core belief really feel this is something you want to go through on a personal level, a competitive level, a participant level, or an idealistic level? Do you believe you're already capable of the race? Do you recognize if you're not?

The belief system must be as equally ready to perform the function as the body. Your belief must be strong enough to push through the low spots, the troubled areas, the stick-points, and the humility of admitting where help or work is needed. Your beliefs must be in order and ready to accept the tasks to fulfill the final goal.

If you believe you'll lose weight, gain strength, consistently keep at it for X number of days and utilize as many areas of your life to achieve those goals, then you will achieve them. If you have doubts, they'll become huge balloons that you won't see past. They'll follow and haunt you because you'll see doubt instead of faith, you'll follow the easier route toward weakness than the challenging road toward strength. Core Beliefs keep you on the Success Path, despite the visibility.

At your Belief Core, you must find some positive light to consistently look toward every day, in the direction of health and fitness. There is no other way. Half-hearted convictions produce half-hearted achievements.

People tend to disagree with this intensity of effort being necessary at every workout, every day. But by being present in every moment, in relaxed attention, the automatic response takes precedence and spontaneity reigns by allowing the body to be comfortable at work, at play, at exercise and at relaxation.

If you train the mind to believe in exercise, to believe in yourself, to believe in the goodness of being attentive in activity and nutrition, the physical will follow, and will lead the body toward better health. You must shape your mind in order to shape your body. Get your thinking in alignment with your beliefs and goals.

To fully invest in a training program, the change must first come in attitude toward exercise. Once your mind begins to believe that exercise is essential, not a task or a curse, but a privilege, then you move into a positive training mode.

As your thoughts take shape, the pace in which you can attain goals accelerates. Do you choose to not set any and go down the lazy river of exercise through the motions of redundant boredom without getting anywhere? Or do you choose to work toward them in focused effort, with "hard work, one hour, each day," until the goals are met?

The belief system you build toward physical fitness will guide you through each workout. You will either exercise this day at this time – or you won't. When you decide that exercise is just as essential for life as food and sleep, your beliefs have a starting point. Do something physically active every single day for 11 days. Consciously think of what you're doing and how you're achieving this first goal. But BELIEVE you will follow through for 11 days and then DO IT! Exercise your belief system to rise up to excellence. Exercise your mind with visualization, mental rehearsal, positive input and feedback.

THE BODY CORE

The Body Core are the parts and the abilities given you at birth and developed through years of various sports and activities, or inactivity. What is your body's condition? Where would you like it to be? Elite athletes can look in the mirror every day and see areas for improvement with complete humility. Why then, can't a man with many numbered weaknesses see something he'd like to move toward in a positive light on a daily basis until it's accomplished?

The Body Core is primarily the heart, the abdominals, the middle and lower back, hip flexors, gluteus and upper legs, front and back. It is your power source, your energy source, your center of gravity, your stabilizing and acceleration system and the storehouse for vital organs. People strong in the core have good posture, few injuries in the lower back and hamstrings, better digestion and greater capability to generate force to the arms and legs.

The very absolute center and most essential aspect of the Body Core is the heart. If you train it both literally and figuratively, you will achieve or gain any goal you set out toward. The stronger you train aerobically, to pump more blood into and from the heart in its most efficient method of transport, the better off your whole system will become.

From the heart, the stomach and organs support, stabilize and respirate the body. The legs, hips and gluteus engage the lower body to propel it into motion in any direction. The arms help to accelerate this directional energy and are enlisted in catching, carrying, reaching, holding, strength, speed and stride. They are powered by the core to deliver explosive energy in many combinations of movement.

By starting with the heart, the core responds with energy emanated from the hub to the extremities, delivering the necessary force, strength and balance to accomplish the activity put before it. The more this Consistent Organized Rehearsal of Exercises is practiced, the sharper and more natural the response. You mentally create what you would like to do with the physical body you have. Is it to run faster, run longer, play sports, build strength, alleviate pain, or change the shape, symmetry and composition of your body? What can you begin to think of as an initial compass point to give you a radius of training?

What does the sport you participate in require? Does it require bulk, speed, flexibility, fast hands, or fast feet? What combinations of attributes will help you not just to participate, but to compete at a higher level of play? As you make this mental assessment, you begin to formulate physical goals.

If it is better health in general that you seek, how strongly do you feel about improving your health wholeheartedly? Do you plan to do just some things and not others, thereby getting just some results and not all? Or will you do all you can to feel better? Believe, simply, that you can do some sort of exercise each day, that you'll implement better nutritional choices daily, and that you will do it for the rest of your life. You will feel the results in clarity, energy, attitude and sleep. You'll be eager to share these new feelings with others and want to learn more to expand the feelings of goodness and health.

Training the Body Core strengthens the extremities as well as the core; training only the extremities weakens the core and adds insult to injury by way of disproportionate development, overtraining and weak links. If all you do is train the body center, the rest of the body will be strong enough to carry you through. When you incorporate exercises that train the Body Core and Core Beliefs, you synchronistically join all aspects of your being into the task at hand.

THE CORE EXERCISES

The Core Exercises are the third aspect of the total core. They are the basis of what you must do as the minimum requirements to compete in your sport. You can learn, apply, and try various methods and movements, but if you concentrate on compound movements which work across multiple joints and muscle groups, you'll be stronger on many planes. The more universally you apply this simple method over the whole body, the better and sooner will be the results, all over your body. The input is equal to the output.

The exercises work best when they follow a specific pattern of training, over an optimum number of weeks, until results taper off. A strictly structured plan without deviation is unproductive and boring. Variety within guidelines keeps you in tune with your body's growing ability to do more, more efficiently, faster, and with less pain.

Our training toolbox is enhanced by familiarity and use. The more we draw from practiced methods on a regular basis, the more apt we are to have each at our disposal, and the discretion to know when to use each one. From the basic fundamentals come the aspects of practice which lead to mastery. No one goes straight to mastery. Therefore, the body must first find its anchor in the core and grow outwardly from there. We each have the same tools to participate in sport and in life. It's what we choose to do with the time and space between that makes the short man the professional basketball player or the one-legged woman an Olympic skier.

From the core group of exercises are the stems into individualized sports. Golfers think the sport alone is enough for exercise. If it means they golf or do nothing, then of course, golf is enough. But not really, they will not improve their game until they do more in preparation for it. Just think if Olympic skiers only ran the course, time after time. The ones who go over and above with their training preparations are always the ones who win. Always. They invent their own ways of getting the highest performance out of their bodies, and time after time, they get it. Going that extra mile means believing something more than your opponents and peers.

Often, the young athlete trains with intensity and passion on the wrong areas, the "show Muscles." They train the arms and chest and sometimes abdominals for the sake of aesthetics, without considering how these muscles work in relation to their sports. There are some who train arms and chest for years on end whose net results are too often torn shoulders and bad backs. The adage, "You're only as strong as your weakest link," is especially true in strength training. Constant favoring of muscle groups and exercises leads to great imbalances and eventually, injury.

After this Core discipline is learned, there will be other things to focus on and to master, and your life will continue on an upward arc rather than a downward spiral. Resolve that it should never be "done." If you learn all the basics of core training, making good movements and good techniques become your habits, you will be able to design a program for any sport you choose. The exercises are comprised of basic standing and mat exercises that can be completed anywhere, and a series of stretches that should be done in order to awaken the muscles to exercise. These core movements should be done daily, before or after a workout, and even without a workout, just done alone. The stretches and the exercises are a very good opportunity to tune in to your limitations. Don't skip any part of them but instead keep trying to perform them better, with greater stability and focus.

11 ESSENTIAL CORE STRETCHES

To stretch is to know your body in a whole new way. You really begin to realize where you are tight and what you must do to alleviate that tightness. You begin to know the landscape of your body, topographically, on many levels. When you recognize an imbalance, you offer counterbalance – you correct, straighten, apply pressure, heat or relieve the contraction with breath, reach, release and rest. Stretching means movements in set patterns on a regular basis. Once stretching is incorporated every day, in classrooms, in homes, in offices; everyone will not only be more limber, but more relaxed, less stressed, and more prone toward happiness!

The set of 11 core stretches, which are essential for keeping the muscles long and the body supple, should optimally be done in this order. Hold each stretch for 11 seconds. Make adjustments in stance or position to keep comfortable.

> _Reach Up_ – from a standing position; reach up through the center of your body to the left, then right, then straight overhead. Anchor the heels.
>
> _Reach Down_ –fold in half and stretch toward your toes, without bouncing or forcing the movement, simply hanging loose toward the floor.
>
> _Downward Facing Dog_ – hands flat on the floor, feet flat, hips high with tailbone
>
> toward the ceiling, spread legs if necessary to push heels to floor.
>
> _Low Hips_ – let your knees sink to the ground, thighs touching the floor, back
>
> arched and chin pulled up toward the ceiling, slow and controlled.
>
> _Kneeling & Reaching_- knees on floor, sit back on heels with arms outstretched forward and head

down between arms, reach forward as you sit back, pressing tops of feet toward the floor to stretch the ankles.

Flat Supermans – lay on your stomach reaching through fingers and toes, like Superman flying flat on the ground, head and neck stretched forward through the crown, reaching simultaneously in both directions.

Hands & Heels – flip to your back and again reach through the hands and heels, pushing out overhead and through your calves to your heels.

Straight Leg Lift – on your back, bend one leg so knee points to ceiling, foot flat on floor; raise opposite leg with knee locked, straight up, as if placing the heel on the ceiling, hold. Release. Repeat on other leg.

Knee To Chest – pull one bent leg in to chest, opposite leg outstretched, hold leg with both arms while raising the head toward knee, touching nose to knee to stretch neck and shoulders. Repeat with other leg.

Two Knees To Chest – leave head down, pull both knees in to chest, flattening hips and shoulders to the floor as much as possible.

Twisting Crossover – release the knees and stretch overhead, then place both hands together and twist upper body toward right while bent right knee goes toward left side. Repeat with opposite arm and leg.

FIVE ESSENTIAL CORE EXERCISES

1.*FOUR SIDED PLANKS*

Begin with the body on the floor, face down on the forearms and knees. Lift the body into a "plank" so only the toes and arms are touching. Keep the abdominals tight, the back and buttocks contracted, the neck straight and hold for 11 seconds in this up position. Return to rest on the floor.

Turn on the left side with left forearm on the floor and the arm bent at 90°. Stack the right foot directly on top of the left, then lift the left side of the body completely off the floor so only the forearm and foot are touching. Keep the right hand flat against the right thigh, the abs, buttocks and lower back tightly contracted and the neck straight. Hold for 11 seconds, then rest.

Turn onto the back with elbows bent under the upper body so the torso is raised diagonally from tailbone to neck. Lift the body in a straight "plank" so the hips rise nearly as high as the chest, with hips, buttocks and back contracted and the neck straight. Hold for 11 seconds, then rest.

Turn on the right side with right forearm on the floor and the arm bent at 90°. Stack the left foot directly on top of the right, then lift the right side of the body completely off the floor so only forearm and foot are touching. Keep the left hand flat against the left thigh, the abs, buttocks and lower back tightly contracted and the neck straight. Hold for 11 seconds, then rest. Repeat for two more rotations to total 3 sets of 11 seconds on each side of the 4-Sided Planks.

A beginner should set their body down between "planks." But to make this more challenging, move from front to side to back to side for 11 seconds per plank without ever dropping the body in between. Other variations include raising the top arm or leg or both arm and leg from the side plank; and raising the abs and buttocks into an inverted "V" from the face down position.

2.*THE POINTER*

Place hands and knees on the floor with back flat and neck straight. The face should be held parallel to the ground. Raise the left leg straight out behind until it is level with the back, toe pointed backward, abs, lower back and buttocks tight. Raise the right arm straight up, fingers pointed forward, until it is level with the shoulder. Stretch through the neck, elongating through the crown of the head. Push through both the toes and fingertips, lengthening the body as long as possible. Hold the arm and leg up for 11 seconds and do not start the count until both are raised. Repeat with the right leg and left arm, rest; then continue for two more rounds on each side for a total of 3 sets.

The advanced version of this move is to begin with only the hands and feet on the ground, the body raised in a high pushup. Spread the legs for a wider base. Raise the left leg as high as possible, then the right arm, striving to reach out in both directions as high and forward as possible while keeping the abs, lower back and buttocks contracted and the neck straight, the face parallel to the floor. Repeat with the opposite arm and leg.

This move must be done slowly and only after practicing the other exercises of core strengthening. There will be a noticeable improvement after a few days of stability training and with this improved stabilization comes more flexibility and endurance.

3.*TWISTING PENDULUM*

Stand with both feet facing forward, hands pressed flat, fingertips together in front of chest. Raise the left leg slightly above the right ankle, balanced against the standing leg. With fingers pointing upward, the chest high, the abs and buttocks tight, turn the hands and shoulders away from the left leg until the hands align with the right hip, while balancing only on the right foot. Turn slowly back to the left until the hands align with the left hip. Keep the elbows raised, the hands pressed together and the foot raised until 11 twists are accomplished. Switch legs and repeat for 11 reps. Do 3 sets of 11 repetitions total for each side.

As core stability and strength increase, raise the foot higher up the standing leg toward the knee, and try to increase speed in the repetitions.

4._FRONT LEG PULL and "V"_

Sit on a mat in an "L" shape, chest lifted, legs straight, toes pointed, wrists even with the hips, fingertips forward, butt on the ground throughout. Tighten abs and lift hips so body forms a straight line. Keeping hips lifted, raise straightened left leg off floor. Hold for a 3 count, lower the left leg and repeat with the right, and then raise both legs. Do 11 reps each - left, right, both for 11 seconds - keeping the body straight. This exercise is a perfect lead-in to the "V."

From the seated position, raise both the arms and legs to balance only on the sit-bones, attempting to touch the toes of both feet with the fingers of both hands, and then settling into a "V," finding balance only on the buttocks. Bring the legs down, above the floor and the arms outstretched, as the starting position. Repeat touches for 11 reps.

5._THE PENDULUM_

Lay flat on the floor on your back, the hips, shoulder blades and entire back except for it's natural curve above the lumbar, touching the floor. Bring both legs straight up as if placing the heels on the ceiling.

Press through the heels. Keep the head down. Place the arms out to the side for balance and attentively roll the shoulders openly toward the floor, palms up. Hold this position for 11 seconds, lengthening the spine toward the head, the arms to the sides and the legs from the hips. Slowly, very slowly, let the feet drop for an 11 count toward the left, then bring them back to center, stabilize, and let them drop to the right in 11 counts. This is one repetition. Rest. Do a total of 11 repetitions, at first, one at a time – center, left and right – and work toward stringing 2, 3, 4, 5, 6, and then all 11 together at once.

"The vision must be followed by the venture. It is not enough to stare up the steps — we must step up the stairs." –Vance Havner

2

<u>HEART</u>
<u>& HANDS</u>

"One Hollows The Clay And Shapes It Into Pots:

In Its Nothingness Consists The Pot's Effectiveness."

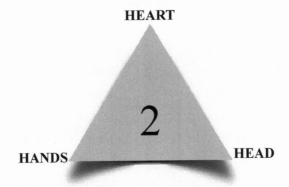

HEART AND HANDS

By "hollowing the clay" of our bodies to shape them to our desired forms, we open the heart and open the hands, literally and figuratively. We reach in each direction of a stretch because our bodies have become huddled and contorted, compressed and distorted by our daily deeds.

What we do with the "clay that shapes the pot" varies according to our talents, ambitions, vision, instruction and application. We are created equal, barring background, deformities or handicaps. We all have the same flesh and bones that are our substances. We each have our own specific, genetic make-up which makes us physically look the way we do, shapes our muscles, and determines the length of our limbs and the strength of our hearts. This is the "nothingness" we begin to shape into something greater.

We open the heart, letting calmness and fresh air to enter and expand its chambers. The fats and processed foods constricting its essential movement and basic operations are allowed to release. The pressure on the organs from bad posture, endless sitting, slouching and gravity itself is changed when reaching high, bending low and stretching out flat on the floor. The "nothingness" there is the space between the arms and legs, between the chest and neck and tailbone as the flat earth grounds you and calms the vibrations of the body to a noticeable hum that lulls the body into the "ahh" you are, laying flat on the floor, mimicking Da Vinci's perfect proportions as you expand in every direction by laying motionless. You arch your body to receive this "nothingness" which really becomes the "effectiveness" your body needs.

Opening the heart and hands to the challenges of the body in exercise movements forms the clay of our flesh. What is taken away, in terms of extraneous equipment and entertainment, are further distractions from the centered focus one needs in exercise. By taking away, we gain. By using our hearts and our hands we are freed to new levels of improved movement.

We take what we have, and through activity, nutrition and environment we develop our abilities and talents. We hollow the clay and shape the pots that are our lives. We add more muscle here, take fat away there, add strength, flexibility, and balance and by this gain speed, endurance, power and longevity. Our "effectiveness" comes from developing what we have to begin with.

The effective "nothingness" is the ability to stop thinking during competition and allow the body to perform automatically. If balance, footwork, stability, strength and flexibility are practiced consistently, play becomes play. The neuroskeletal system responds to the stimulus put upon it, compensating at various angles, planes and leverages with speed, force and focus.

We all begin with the same set of tools; our bodies that we were born with, our brains and hearts to become whatever we set out to become, and our hands and legs to get us wherever we move toward. We each have "Heart and Hands."

START WITH THE HEART

The first thing to identify us before birth is the ultrasound of our heartbeat. That is all that defines us. It identifies us as a human in our mother's womb. That is where we started. The Latin origin for the word "Core" is "Heart".

As we begin any exercise program or workout regimen we should also start with the heart to make sure it is strong enough to handle the stress we plan to put before it. By learning to target and train the heart for ultimate efficiency, you can increase many areas of the whole physical system by concentrating on just one. The stronger the heart, the stronger the whole system you can build around it. If it is weak, so too will you be.

The benefits of beginning a cardiovascular program are numerous. The first goal is to raise your heart rate through aerobic exercise. Walking exercises your lungs and circulatory system, bringing more oxygen and blood to the brain and heart tissue, which improves mood, alertness, and stimulates the release of endorphins, the "feel good" hormones. By releasing endorphins it combats depression and elevates mood in general, along with well-being and self-esteem through accomplishment, confidence and self –sufficiency.

Walking is also the most available form of exercise, it can be performed virtually anywhere, has the lowest incidence of injury and enhances mobility. Anyone can do it, from the obese 8 year old to the ailing 80 year old. It keeps blood pressure normal, enriches the heart and arteries, lowers cholesterol, increases bone strength and burns excess calories in the most beneficial, least taxing way.

Other positive side effects are that sleep improves and the nervous system gets a workout by stimulating balance and stability when moving your arms rapidly in a rhythmic, cadenced tempo. Once this simple exercise is incorporated into a daily regimen, it often leads to other forms of cardiovascular training.

The maximum heart rate is basically calculated as the number 220 minus your age, multiplied by 70-85% to find your optimal heart rate zone. There are other more precise ways to gauge optimum heart rate, but this is a simple formula that works. For example: a 30 year old would be 220-30 = 190. 70% of that would be 190 x .70 = 133 heartbeats per minute. To exercise in a higher zone, multiply by .80 for 152 heartbeats and let that be the upper levels per minute. The simplest way to check your heart rate is to count your pulse for 6 seconds and multiply that by 10, i.e., 15 pulses x 10 = 150 heartbeats per minute.

Keeping the heart in this zone for a 22 – 33 minute period will begin to show immediate benefits. If it's too hard to sustain that rate, that's all the more reason to keep working at it consistently, but at a slower pace. If it's easy to achieve, try taking it to 85% of your maximum and attempt to sustain that level for 44 – 55 minutes. This is the cardio-effect. This is exercising the heart to handle the workload you plan to put on it with exercise and weights.

Start with the heart. A healthy heart will garner far-reaching effects by burning excess calories and conditioning the whole body to work more efficiently. Exercising the heart in an aerobic capacity will put the body in motion as well as the blood. The less resistance the body has internally, by keeping a healthy heart system, the more performance you will get out of the graduated aspects of training.

This is the something from nothing the poem refers to; you may not be doing anything more than walking, but by doing it with a plan and concentrated effort, you are effectively causing the body to change by accepting or rejecting the exercise, and compensating further progress.

By beginning with the heart and hands we assure our bodies and minds of exactly what we start with. Going through a week of freehand exercises will get the body acclimated to exercise, will point out weaknesses, imbalances and strengths, and will incorporate a discipline that accepts no exceptions or excuses because the body and gravity are all that's required to begin.

This is what Nike meant when it said, "Just do it" The effective nothingness is the ability to stop thinking during competition and allow the body to perform automatically. To shape yourself for a particular sport is to fashion your personal vehicle that drives you to your chosen destination.

START WALKING!

You want to exercise, change your physique, improve your game, time, swing, etc. But you don't know where or how to start. Start where all great athletes and thinkers throughout history started – walk. Yes, walk. Not exactly what you expect to hear for high performance training. But babies walk before they run, animals learn balance before mastering speed, and you must take time to THINK about what you expect to get out of training and how high a level of fitness you hope to attain by paying attention to simple signs inherent in your present condition.

So walk, but walk with purpose and careful attention to your gait. Are your shoulders even? Do your hips overswing or hold back your stride? How about your arms, your neck, the direction of your feet; do they move with the forward motion of your body or hang limp? Have you ever thought about this simple exercise and how it reveals inconsistencies or injuries?

This is the one exercise you have no excuse to participate in? Walking trails and mall participation programs are proliferating. There is space on the beach, in the neighborhood, in the park, throughout schools and wherever you may find yourself. Even in a hotel with no other outlet except staircases, along with high-rise offices and apartment buildings, you can walk anywhere, any time.

WALK

A cardiovascular program can be started easily by walking 15 minutes from your house or office, turning around and walking back in 15 minutes or less. On the next day, make it to the same place, and then go further. Do the return in the same 15 minutes. Continue this for the first 3 days, adding distance to the trip out and speed to the trip back.

On the fourth through sixth days go out a full 20 minutes and repeat the pattern of longer trips out, faster paces back. The seventh, eighth and ninth days are increased to 30 minutes out, 30 minutes back, with the same graduated intensity as the previous days. It may require running to meet the times, so an easy pattern for a suburban neighborhood is to run a block, then walk a block, and continue alternating until you get to stringing the runs 2, 3, and 4 blocks together.

Days 10 and 11 do a full run/walk pattern of 30 minutes out and 30 back. Notice how much further you go on your route by running it. With this, you will then have a 60-minute program in place that will constitute your 3-day per week cardiovascular program. Fast walking can also be substituted in place of running.

PUT YOUR HEART INTO IT

This conditioning is the most important thing to do from the outset of any exercise program. Once you get the heart working efficiently, a noticeable feeling will come into your life. You will see the everyday things which made you winded are no longer difficult, the stairs no longer daunting, lifting boxes or playing with the kids in the yard, easier. Your complexion will be rosier, your well-being in general will improve; and especially notice this, you will recruit others to join in this program, you will want to share the good feelings and positive benefits with someone else, not only as a companion, but because you care about them. You will lead others to health by walking.

JUMPING ROPE

This is an advanced form of cardiovascular training. It develops speed, timing, explosiveness, superb aerobic endurance and coordination. With jump-roping, you burn more calories per minute because both your hands and your legs are moving, coupled with the jumping motion, so that 10 to 20 minutes of jumping rope seem like twice the time running.

Find an adequate space, a comfortable pace, and skip. Music helps to establish an even tempo. Try whatever variation of steps that work for you. If you must jump with both feet in a double jump, fine; if you must use a running style, with one foot following the other over the rope, good; if you use a rocking jump with one leg in front of the other while rocking forward and back, good for you. Just avoid running out of the gate like a horse in a race. Calmly find a tempo that you can sustain for at least 11 minutes.

To work up to 11 minutes at a time, start with 2 minutes on, 1 minute off, 2 on, 1 off, until 11 total minutes elapse. Then get to 3 on, 1 off. Then 4 on, 1 off, and finally 5 on, 1 off, and 5 on to total 11 minutes. The next progression is 11 minutes in a row nonstop. Once this is accomplished, simply add 1 minute per workout until you can sustain 33 minutes straight as the ultimate aerobic goal, taking 1 minute breaks when necessary. Another easy way to break 33 minutes down is to do 10 minutes on, 1 off, 10 on, 1 off, until the 33 total are accomplished, and then proceed to 33 straight.

At first, you legs will ache as if someone were holding them down, as if your feet were stuck in muck up to the ankles. Your quads will feel heavy and ready to burst with each breath. Your arms will weaken with every turn of the jump rope. Just lifting your feet off the ground will be the initial goal. Your focus will shift from the rope, to the floor, to the clock. You count turns. You miss steps. The rope burns as it hits the calves on missed jumps. This is the first 6 minutes for the first 3 days.

By the second week the tempo will be there. You'll find balance. The twist and the jump become one. You are able to focus on the music, the tempo of the rope, your breath. It still hurts. It still burns, but now it's tolerable. Now you can truly see a way to the end of the 6 minutes.

Within a month you'll be up to 11 minutes, with periodic rests of a minute or less. Your heart will beat 60 times stronger. Your legs will feel lighter. Your steps like a dancer. Your arms in even cadence to the rope going around. Sweat will pour off of you like pounds. You'll be astounded by how little effort creates such great results. Foot speed, heartbeat, balance, breathing all play out with this one simple exercise.

The added benefits of jumping rope are tighter calves, hamstrings, quadriceps and butt, and burning more calories for your time. Foot and ankle strength are enhanced, body balance, core strength, lower back firmness and shoulder strength are also affected with this simple exercise. Packing a rope into a suitcase provides an aerobic workout no matter where you travel.

It's not for everyone because if bodyweight lingers toward obese, the stress on the bones and joints is greater than the benefits. But as bodyweight decreases and cardiovascular capacity increases, it is a good exercise to progress toward in addition to, or as a replacement to, a walk/run program. Small trampolines also offer similar benefits, but are less portable and more of an expense.

USE YOUR HANDS

Use the equipment necessary for every sport and activity that you currently have and always will have, YOUR BODY. Use your bodyweight as its own resistance when you begin a strength training program. Once you learn how to add repetitions and sets to a foundation based on good form, you'll learn how to build a program that disciplines your body in every area, alleviating weaknesses and building strength upon strength for better athletic performance, better health, longevity and lifelong activity. And you'll learn how to get all you need from the environment already available to you.

A step, a floor, a pull-up bar, a chair, a resistance ball, a track, a gym, a pool, a park, a playground all offer areas where a little knowledge, imagination, discipline and commitment can increase your level of fitness 110% from where it currently is.   Sometimes the simplest training can teach us the most about our bodies. A push up teaches us uniformity, balance, strength, discipline, pacing, endurance, stability and a way to see measurable gains on a timely basis. As long as you have your hands you can build upper body strength.

Deliberate, repetitive, identical, one-right-after-the-other–moves, train the muscles and also the neuroskeletal system. Begin with as many repetitions as you can, until you can perform 11 perfectly. By holding the contraction and extension fully, you're sending serious signals to your nerve fibers. You're giving your muscles a predetermined "groove." The shape they take is determined by your will, vision and ability to concentrate fully in each repetition.

THE PUSH UP

The pushup is hard to match for challenging upper body strength. As a basic daily exercise, the first challenge will be to do a set of 11 repetitions. This exercise works the front of the body across the chest and shoulders, the triceps, upper back and even the stomach through enhanced core stability.

There are other variations to be done for specific strengthening regimens, such as incline, decline, staggered and additional resistance or apparatus pushups with the swissball or Bosu, but the basic pushup is a core "hand" movement which measures progress as well as continually challenging you as the repetition range increases. Measurable progress is evident as each day you can do more repetitions with stricter form, and then more sets with shorter rest periods.

BEGINNER PUSH UP

If you haven't done pushups, or have not done them in a long time, it's best to start with the knees on the floor, hands under the shoulders, fingers pointing straight ahead. Lower your chest to the floor by bending only your elbows, keeping the lower back and stomach firmly rigid, the neck and face looking slightly ahead. Do as many as you can in this way, up to 11 repetitions. If you must break it down into smaller sets of 4,4,3 or 6,5 reps, do it until you get all the 11 repetitions in one smooth, perfect-form set. You will total 33 repetitions for this workout, beginning with the 3 sets of 11 repetitions, broken down as necessary to complete all the reps.

INTERMEDIATE PUSH UP

The next challenge is to take the intensity up by doing regular, military style push-ups with only the toes and hands touching the floor. Again, the stomach and lower back stay rigid, the neck and face straight ahead in a forward gaze. Begin each set in this upright position and accomplish as many as possible before dropping to the knees to complete the set. A grand total of 33 is the first goal in 3 sets of 11 repetitions.

ADVANCED PUSH UP

Initially, this set can be broken down in any combination to total 55. Ultimately, the long-term goal is for 55 strict, straight pushups in a minute or less. This can be broken down into sets of 33, 22 or 22, 22, 11; but ultimately, being able to accomplish 55 push-ups in 60 seconds is the end goal for this exercise.

On a daily basis, move to 5 sets of 11 in a workout, periodically challenging yourself to performing 55 in one set with one rest. Keep in mind that form matters more than number, getting through the sets with complete range of motion and as good of form as possible, first in small increments to meet the repetition goals, then to meet the higher numbers. It's actually better to stop in guided amounts rather than doing all you can until you drop, every set.

PULL UPS

The pull-up is the second hand movement that incorporates all the upper body muscles from the hip flexors upward in its vertical pull against gravity, using only body-weight as resistance. Do not be discouraged if a first attempt accomplishes only one half of one repetition. When this movement is mastered and 11 or more in a set are the normal range of repetitions, you can be sure that your upper body strength is balanced and intact.

If a chinning bar is not available, start with a thick broomstick across two chairs, with your body on the floor on your back. Grasp the stick in an overhand grip outside shoulder width, and pull the chest to the bar. This is not as effective as a conventional pull up, but until a bar is available, it will suffice.

Variations, such as the "chin up", done with palms facing toward you, places the stress more on the biceps and the front of the body. The "pull up," done with palms facing away from you on the bar, stresses all the major back muscles as well as the rear shoulders, trapezius, biceps, triceps and forearms. Grip strength is also enhanced.

It is important to train from the start in a full hanging position, with arms completely extended. Half reps in this movement are encouraged simply because, when beginning this movement, that's usually all anyone can accomplish. All movements, with few exceptions, should be performed from full extension to full contraction. But continue attempting to get farther up and closer to the bar with as many reps as possible. Total 11 repetitions in as many sets as it takes, even if it's initially 11 sets of 1 rep. Ultimately, perform 3 sets of 11 repetitions as a complete pull up workout.

One variation with a regular pull-up bar or one which hangs in a doorway, is to place a folding chair under the bar with the back of it, away from you and the seat under your body. Place one foot on the seat and the other on the back of the chair. While hanging on to the bar with the feet in place underneath on the chair; boost yourself up with your legs by stepping on the back of the chair with the other foot balanced on the seat. This will assist you until you can master a pull up on your own without assistance.

DIPS

A dip works the lower and outer portion of the chest, the triceps and the shoulders. It is a primary bodyweight exercise for gaining upper body strength and for shaping the chest on its outer edges. Dips, done correctly, through their full range of motion, provide strength for movements such as the bench press and row. They work on the vertical plane, complimenting the Pushup on the horizontal plane. Their direct stimulus of the chest and triceps make them an excellent shaping movement.

Begin with the balance of bodyweight focused rearward - the legs crossed or hanging diagonally backward, chin up, hands in a grip at or inside shoulder width. This works the triceps, trapezius and upper back.

When the balance is focused forward - chin to chest, hands in a narrow grip, legs angled to the front of the body -the main areas exercised are the chest, the upper, outer latissimus (back) and front deltoids.

The best stimulation, therefore, comes from a combination of sets of a forward focus, alternated with sets with a rearward focus. The dip is essential to create power in the fully extended regions of the chest as well as arm power for movements or activities which require a forward thrust such as blocking, sprinting from blocks, reaches in volleyball or basketball, grappling, swimming strokes and any other sports which require the arms to move both quickly away from the body and retract fully toward it.

Total 11 repetitions in as many sets as it takes, even if it's initially 11 sets of 1 rep. Ultimately, perform 3 sets of 11 repetitions as a complete dip workout. It would also be good to counter your pull-ups with sets of dips in between.

USE YOUR LEGS

The legs have more muscle fibers than any other bodypart. They are the longest muscles in the body. The legs are the only bodypart we can work solely, and gain muscle mass throughout the rest of the body, because that many fibers are fired. Leg strength is paramount to any and every activity. When a child walks their first steps, it's a major turning point in their lives. When an old person loses mobility, it's a major detriment to their lives.

Leg training is easy to find yet often taxing to perform. The entire respiratory system, muscular system, balance system and energy reserves are pushed to extremes. We get out of breath from the demands of our legs. Our heart pounds resoundingly when our legs are working hard. But when our legs are in shape, we can seemingly go on for hours at our activities.

It is important to train them on as many planes as they work. We must lunge, we must squat, we must jump, and we must move laterally. And, we must be flexible enough to move through all the motions and activities required to stimulate them.

THE LUNGE

This simple lower body movement is essential not only to every person in any form of athletics, but to the beginning and intermediate exerciser as well. It is the essential lower body exercise. The lunge improves acceleration, braking, directional stability, core stability, cardiovascular endurance and literally works every muscle of the leg, from the tiny balancing muscles of the foot and ankle, up through the front and rear calves and their overlapping insertions, to the stabilizing muscles of the knee and its critical tendons, then continuing upward through the thigh and hamstrings, the inner and outer stabilizing muscles on the sides of the legs, right up to the gluteus and into the external oblique, serratus and abdominal muscles, the core. Posture and balance are improved with this movement, as well as accelerating the heartrate.

Because so many muscles are involved, performing the lunge in its simplest forward and back form completely taxes the cardiovascular system. The numerous variations of steps, directions and apparatus challenge the lower body system further for specific stimulation; but as an overall, daily, lower body movement, the stepping or stationary lunge cannot be beat.

STATIONARY LUNGES

Begin with both feet even, shoulder width apart. Step forward with the left foot until the right trailing leg forms a 90° angle with the knee toward the ground and the leading leg forming a 90° angle with the upper leg straight and the knee NOT extended over the toe. Keep the shoulders over the hips, the hands off the knees, chin up and arms at the sides.

Stay in this stationary lunge, performing 11 bends on the left, taking the knee to the floor for each repetition. Step back to the starting position, then out with the right foot leading and perform 11 stationary lunges on that leg. The end goal is to perform 3 x 22 on each leg in one workout.

ALTERNATING-STEPS LUNGES

Begin with both feet even, shoulder width apart. Step forward with the left foot until the rear leg forms a 90° angle with the knee toward the ground and the leading leg forms a 90° angle with the upper leg straight and the knee NOT extended over the toe. Keep the shoulders over the hips, the hands off the knees, chin up and arms at the sides. Push off the left foot to return to the starting position.

Step forward and back, alternating legs, until 22 total repetitions are done, 11 per leg. Land on the heel of the foot on the forward step and push from the ball of the foot to return rather than the toes when getting back to the even position. Stay as erect as possible for better balance and to utilize the stabilizing muscles on the hips and lower back. At first you may not be able to step out very far, but keep striving to "lunge" further forward in each successive step.

SQUATS

These are also a necessity for any leg development program, every sport, everyone wishing to add strength, speed, shape, or mobility to their athletic and everyday life. They need to be done with a complete range of motion, which must first be practiced "free-hand," without additional weight or equipment.

Begin with feet in "ready" stance, under the shoulders, toes pointed straight ahead. This is the stance one assumes for sports, like the tennis, baseball and volleyball player in "readiness" for play; a slight crouch with knees bent and pointed forward, shoulders and hips squared. For balance, allow the arms to raise upward while the body descends into the squat, through the glutes, hamstrings, calves and quadriceps. Lower your body as far as possible toward the floor while keeping the knees pointed straight ahead and the heels on the floor. The inability the keep the heels down is initially a matter of lacking flexibility in the ankles and balance in the core. With time, concentration and practice, while proceeding in a slow, controlled movement through the full range of motion, a complete squat will be possible.

Perform 3 sets of 11 repetitions. As you get stronger, challenge yourself in the middle set to do 22 repetitions; then, two of the three sets for 22 reps; and ultimately, 3 sets of 22 repetitions.

"LEGS BE REAL"

No other training is as important as leg training. None is more neglected. When done consistently, the depth of the pain fades and the feeling of "solidness" is a constant that leads with every step. It's important to stretch the legs after and even during every workout. Blood flow to and from the heart to the working legs is sometimes so great that it can cause nausea if too much work is done too rapidly. So go slowly and completely with as full a range of motion as possible in all these leg movements. At first it may seem like an insurmountable challenge to perform the exercises, but once the routine is incorporated into a workout regimen, every other area will be stronger and more solid.

USE YOUR HEAD

Being fit and healthy is something that should be a given in everyone's life. To pursue better fitness is possible even from a healthy, fit state. A byproduct of this continual vigilance to a higher quality of health is a sharpened mind. Thinking of what will be done each day to enhance the body should come alongside thoughts of what you'll eat for lunch. The reading of stock market reports, box scores, entertainment news and headlines should include exercise tips and the latest health research. To balance your lifestyle is to include healthy aspects as a necessity, without becoming obsessions. You need not try every exercise, just as you need not buy every pair of shoes.

People often have the misconception that playing a sport will put them into shape, when they should arrive at their sport in their best condition to expect the best performance. The seasonal tennis player, golfer, softball player or skier gets off the couch only in time to make it to the game. Their out of shape body is thrown further out of whack like a clay ball tossed against a wall. Small pains turn to micro tears, turn to pulled muscles, turn to full blown injuries which often go untreated and end up emanating throughout the body as compensating injuries, and the actual source of the pain is lost amidst many imbalances.

A skier who strengthens his core, his back, his legs, his cardiovascular capacity, his focus, his flexibility, and his nutrition, has a much better time skiing both competitively and recreationally because his agility, stamina and self-confidence allow him to make the most of any conditions and situations. The training contains all aspects. The "nothingness" means "no-thing" has gone untrained.

As long as we use our heads, we can find fun and functional ways of exercising. How can people complain when there are as many challenges to keep you fit as there are to make you sick? Active involvement in your health brings active results. An active body gets better at being active, by being active. A sedentary body becomes more sedentary. When something becomes immobile, it first breaks down, then rots.

F.R.E.E.H.A.N.D.

F *REQUENCY* - It is necessary to set an every day record-pattern to success.

R *EPETITION* – Each one cuts the groove in the muscle deeper, delineating it.

EX*AGGERATION* –Bring attention to form and function through
exaggerated movement.

E *FFICIENCY* – This saves time, motion and utilizes energy in a positive manner.

H *ABIT* – Make a goal of creating new, positive, healthy habits consistently.

A *TTENTION* – Put the mind in the muscle and the muscle in the mind.

N *UMBERS* – Complete what you set out to accomplish, do every repetition.

D *ETERMINATION* – You will, you must and you CAN do this. Be unwavering.

F *REQUENCY*

This set of exercises must be performed daily for the first 11 days – every exercise, every day. Do not cut corners, do not jump from one exercise to the next or skip any in between. Do each of them every day for 11 days and you are more than halfway to a new habit, which kicks in around 20 days. You will see measurable progress on a day-to-day basis. Some days will be easier than others. Some will find one movement consistently easy and others surprisingly hard. By that 11th day you'll show a marked improvement in all of them. You may even be looking for your own ways to make them more challenging.

This daily frequency can be applied to any one of these exercise regimens. But if you begin with this first one and build consistently from it, you will have learned to incorporate a whole series of movements and tools into your repertoire from which your mind and body can draw from. Creative ways of doing the same old things will keep the brain fit as well as the brawn, so exercise the mind as well.

R *EPETITION*

Every exercise is based on 11 repetitions or a number divisible by 11. This is simply to do 10% more than anyone else. That one extra repetition every set of every exercise guarantees you're doing over and above the 10 that most other workouts require. It is also insurance in case one or more of the repetitions were sloppy or halfhearted. Do 22 when alternating left and right, 11 per side.

Every movement should mimic the previous one. This way, the muscle follows a "groove," a "line" which defines and separates the bodypart from the corresponding one with definitive "cuts." It's what brings out the separation in a bodypart that makes it noticeable even when in a relaxed position. When beginning this program it is important to try to get through as many repetitions with proper form before giving in or breaking down. Even squeezing out one-half repetitions is encouraged because you're telling your body you are not giving it to weakness, you are dead set on strength.

E *XAGGERATION*

All these exercises require an exaggerated execution to allow the form to reach deeply into the movement, and to register deeply in the brain and nervous system. This helps get a better "feel" for every movement, for which muscles are working and how they mesh together and support one another in supporting the body.

Hold a fully extended position to feel the insertions on the ends of the muscles; hold in a fully contracted position to infuse the muscle with blood and to feel the midsection of it. Exaggerate by going beyond the range of motion in a controlled move, but always do it with concentration and control and not recklessness. If it is too easy to perform any one exercise, do super-slow movements to feel your way through the sets, which further ingrains the infusion of muscle fibers.

E *FFICIENCY*

The shortest distance between two points is a straight line. Efficiency of movement is important because you save time and energy in getting from point A to point B by doing it within the body's natural guidelines of movement and not incorporating other areas that only take away from the energy of what you're doing. Small examples of efficiency would be to keep the head in place doing a set rather than shaking it, lifting it or swinging the arms wildly for balance when the balance really comes from settling the body and feeling where the balance needs to be. When doing leg exercises, the upper body should stay solidly in place, not rocking or flailing. On a move like pull ups or dips, the torso should stay firmly solid throughout the whole core.

H *ABIT*

Creating new healthy habits to replace unhealthy, old habits is as easy as opening your refrigerator. Put cut up celery, carrots, green pepper and fruit chunks within reach on the top shelf. While you're trying to decide what to snack on, snack on them. Replace candy dishes with raw almonds, walnuts and cashews. Every time you walk past the water fountain, stop for a drink. Stop yourself at one serving of anything.

While watching TV, do a set of pushups, sit-ups or lunges during commercials. You will not get up to go to the refrigerator once you've become invigorated with energy from these simple exercises. Sit on the floor and do a series of stretches, then watch someone join you. A bad habit is easier to break when immediately replaced with a good habit or reinforcing behavior. Make rewards a positive thing rather than another bad habit. Don't' reward yourself with ice cream for accomplishing your cardio routine.

Habits are easy to incorporate into your lifestyle. It takes roughly 20 days to replace an old habit with a new one. Done conscientiously, with the realization that you're doing something beneficial and paying attention to how good you're feeling, will ingrain it that much faster into your life, and will soon be the automatic choice.

A *TTENTION*

Each new thing in these workouts should be felt for all they're worth. As simple as they seem, as elementary as they are, they offer your body new avenues to strength. The more attention you bring to the exercise you're attempting, the greater the benefit, no matter how minuscule or mundane the movement may be. When the mind is focused on the body, and this feeling registers immediately with the nervous system, the benefit is greatly increased over the haphazard, lackadaisical attempts of going through the motions. By bringing attention to the body, the body responds and gives results in direct proportion to the energy, with corresponding energy. It's like the difference between really laying in to give a kiss and simply accepting one. The difference in intensity completely determines the results.

N *UMBERS*

Doing all the reps, all the sets and all the exercises are of paramount importance at this stage of the game. Do not slack on the numbers. Do not think by adding one to the first set pads you from the subsequent sets. You do 11 so that at least 10 are good. If all 11 are good, that's to your benefit. The numbers matter. The minutes matter. The time you spend on your health regimen matters and the attention you bring to the exercises makes the difference in achieving results, or not. But do not fall into the trap of thinking just because all the numbers were accomplished that you can slack on intensity, form, efficiency and attention. Conversely, do not get so hung up on the numbers that you're putting your body in jeopardy of injury by sloppily accomplishing the given repetitions. Do the sets with conscientious consideration, with feeling and feedback, taking small breaks along the way to succeed in performing the given number of repetitions. The numbers matter, but not if you're just going through the motions to get them.

D ETERMINATION

This is doable. Your health is more important than any other matter, this day, and every day for the rest of your life. Determination makes the difference between being a pawn to outside negative influences on your life and taking a proactive approach which puts you in charge of how healthfully you spend your life. Be positive that the foods, stresses, air and energy that go through your body are what you want in it and not controlled by someone else, nor outside, extraneous circumstances.

Your determination is the anchor to which you fasten your fitness program. If it drifts, so will you. Let your determination be the guidepost to which you focus your physicality, just as you would with material, work or monetary goals. Be determined to get this aspect of your life in order and watch how quickly and easily the rest of your life aligns, with added vitality, enjoyment and healthy perspective.

__Freehand:__ Basic movements and exercises done without additional apparatus that enable you to work out anywhere at any time without the need for specialized equipment nor excuses.

SO, BE CHILDLIKE

This Heart and Hands approach is a Simple Structured Training system which allows you to invest yourself fully into a workout program that challenges the body with compound movements which call upon groups of muscles to work in a synchronistic manner, adding strength, balance and tone to anyone's body in a safe, controlled escalation of exercises. From this you can graduate to a strength training program with additional weights and equipment.

Remember the analogy to being an infant; the heart develops first, our strength is vital to every aspect from that first breath to our last; the brain is hungry and stimulated, everything is new to the mind, taken in with wonder and attention; the hands and legs are of paramount importance for locomotion and discovery. Use your heart and hands in your approach to exercise with an ambitious hunger for more. Learn, try, experiment, pay attention, and push yourself to new levels of freedom by taking hold of your fitness.

"There is no shortcut. Victory lies in overcoming obstacles every day."

3

<u>BASICS</u>

"One Cuts Out The Doors And Windows

To Make The Chamber: In Their

Nothingness Consists

TheChamber'sEffectiveness"

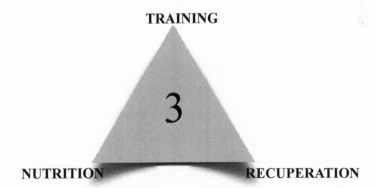

TRAINING

3

NUTRITION   **RECUPERATION**

THE BASICS ARE THE BUILDING BLOCKS

By "cutting out the doors and windows" of our body chamber with the basic tools of exercise, we begin to see what's possible in changing specific aspects of the physique. We begin to see weaknesses and we then take them away with discipline, attention and optimal exercises. What is taken away now serves for "effectiveness," by means of a lighter, leaner, better balanced, more supple, yet stronger, interconnected and synchronistic body.

If a weakness is present and we learn how to eliminate it, the "effectiveness" of the body is enhanced by what is no longer there. If a weakness is known and not addressed, not dealt with or ignored, its presence is then the limiting effect, and this limitation becomes the Achilles heal of our athleticism. Yet, even if it's addressed but not fully remedied, at least something was done to take it away and the mind and body are stronger from the effort.

THE BASICS TRINE

TRAINING / NUTRITION / RECUPERATION

The three main aspects of the Basic program are the Training itself, which should involve both activity in the sport of your participation, and training to counter any weaknesses which need addressing; proper Nutrition with a wide variety of foods and sources of energy to draw from, positive to your sport and lifestyle; and adequate Recuperation, which means resting the muscle groups for adequate periods and also resting the whole body properly. No matter what the regimen is, no matter what sport, what goal, what result you're after, these 3 aspects must be in place for any and every program to work.

Tennis, triathlon, swimming, speed skating, skiing, bodybuilding, golf - each have a recommended set of exercises that are beneficial to that particular sport and are the basic components every participant should master.

But none of these particular activities will be properly ingrained into your consciousness until you physically get out on the field and participate. You can read about them and analyze them all you want; get every video ever made on the subject, consult every expert; but it means nothing until you get your body into the game and experience it firsthand.

Participation in the sport obviously goes hand in hand with Training for the sport. Do the required stretches, warm ups, plyometric moves, weight training, flexibility exercises and mental rehearsal and your body will register a well-rounded repertoire of intuitive experience before you even get to the field.

Once on the field, pay attention to how the body moves, what you use, any limitations felt, the strengths noted, and what it takes to reach "flow," a comfort level where you are in and of the game rather than fighting it to get results. Training encompasses mind, body and spirit and if attention to one or two components is lacking, so too will the results.

Proper Nutrition is the most sensible way to involve the internal/mental Basic aspect. Eating right requires mental discipline and will give your body the results you seek by having the proper energy available at appropriate times. Food is a drug and each type delivers its own energy either for action, strength, explosiveness, recuperation, endurance, repair; and too often, nothing, no nutritional value whatsoever. This is also known as the proverbial "empty calories." Finding what helps and eliminating the "nothing" foods is a huge part of everyone's life, not just the athlete's.

The third aspect, Recuperation, is often one of the most overlooked components for optimal training. If you are sore, or tired, or hung over, or overfed, a tendency to let focus drift occurs because mentally, you may feel there is always another day. You let your body down with inadequate rest, you let your mind down with inadequate discipline, and you let your goals down because you've chosen to be one step further rather than one step closer to a goal.

There are certain things that can be done every day toward your sport or discipline and certain things that should only be done with 48 hours rest, and sometimes more. Intuition and knowing your own body and its abilities only comes with consistent attention and feedback. You must know when to rest it, and when to talk yourself out of the pain and into the training room to massage the body with blood flow and flexibility.

Full recuperation is also a must, to enable the body to bounce back and often launch into a new level of physicality with greater insights and energy and a fully restored focus that comes from stepping back once in a while to observe, meditate and reevaluate approaches or disciplines.

TRAINING BASICS

You are cutting out the doors and windows of your body by refining your moves to suit your particular goals. If you are bodybuilding or sculpting, you add more shape in one area, take away bulk in another. The spaces between constitute all that needs to remain.

The Training Basics apply to all sports, all bodies. This is what building strength is all about. If you learn only these basics and practice them consistently, you will benefit, mind and body, and improve your sport as a result. If you're going to do something repeatedly for a better part of your life, you'd better learn what's safe, as well as comfortable, and what it could possibly do to your body from a structural standpoint, in addition to learning how to prevent injuries rather than repairing breakdowns.

Do you know anyone who complains of wrists or elbows or shoulders or back or knees or hips or feet, and seem to go on this endless circular ride of ailments while letting you know where they are every step of the way? They're like a child on a merry go round, waving each time they pass by, only not quite so happy. You know them when you see them at work, the ones you don't dare ask, "How are you doing?"

"Oh, my elbow, I fell on it the other day because my knee gave out, that's how I got this big gash on my head... Other than that, I'm doing OK! ... I started exercising. I got this ab thingy, it works great... but now my back is killing me..."

The sad part is, we all know someone like that. Walking two extra parking spaces isn't really "incorporating an exercise program." "A burger (hold the mayo), medium fries (instead of supersize) and "a Diet Coke" isn't really cutting calories. It's playing a fools game with food choices, and everyone always sees the fool for what he is, except the fool himself.

Training Basics means all aspects of the physical body are given equal, balanced attention, alleviating weaknesses, accepting but not over-accentuating strengths, and focusing during favorite movements as much as during those less favorable. Everyone must exercise arms, legs, chest, back, butt, shoulders, abdominals, neck, feet, forearms, flexibility, balance, endurance, form, breath, lungs and discipline; everyone, athlete or non.

So! How many aspects have you worked today? Yesterday? Pretty overwhelming? Not really. By laying down a plan and systematically doing a little each day, combining compound movements with isolation moves, prioritizing weaknesses over favoritism and sticking to that plan, will assure better balance not only in the physical body but also in the lifestyle you inhabit.

THE BASIC EXERCISES

THE BENCH PRESS / CHEST

This is the number one upper body chest exercise. It is a compound movement involving the arms, shoulders, back and chest as well as the three joints of the wrist, elbow and shoulder. With its many variations of angles and hand positions, the stresses put on the chest are varied and critical to building upper body strength. Done explosively, it adds power to strength.

Changing the hand grip, from wide to narrow and other points between, will help to mechanically align the body to the most beneficial placement for stimulation. But for just starting out, use one grip consistently to pinpoint the feeling in the proper position across the chest.

Initially, use a medium width grip, just outside the shoulders, with the elbows facing down rather than out. Bring the bar to the bottom edge of the chest line, breathing in as the bar descends, touching the bar all the way to the chest and holding the breath through the hardest explosion of the movement, then exhaling as the arms straighten at their apex. Make every repetition consistent, keeping the back, head and tailbone down on the bench and feet flat on the floor throughout the sets.

Perform 4 sets of 11 repetitions, adding weight if you get all 11, dropping weight if you don't.

THE OVERHEAD ROPE PULL - TRICEPS

This move activates the long heads of the triceps, which are the longest, strongest muscles of the arms, more than any other movement. It also works the middle and outer heads of the triceps. This triple activation will happen only if you drive the hands straight forward with the rope at the top of the movement, rather than any outward turning or bending of the wrists. Separating the rope at extension pushes the stress from the long heads of the triceps to the outer, smaller heads, so avoid the impulse. It is crucial to keep the elbows above the head, the face parallel to the floor and the abs and lower back engaged for stability, with one foot forward for balance.

Face the weight stack with hands on the rope at waist level. Pull down on the stack and pivot away 180° stepping one leg forward of the other, simultaneously ducking the head and raising the arms. Bend only at the elbows to reach back as far as possible without changing the arm position, then straighten the arms to full extension while keeping the rest of the body still. Perform 4 sets of 11 repetitions, adding weight if you get all 11, dropping weight if you don't.

THE BARBELL ROW - BACK

These work the upper, middle and lower back with different stresses on the width and thickness of the muscles by varying the grip. The back is a large muscle group requiring much energy, therefore it should be done early in the workout. Holding the bar with the palms up activates the front face of the latissimus muscles, adding thickness. Turning the hands to palms down activates more stress across the width of the back. So alternating palms up/ palms down, set by set, will be the most beneficial approach to add both width and thickness to the back.

Grasp the barbell outside shoulder width, bend the knees slightly, lift the barbell from the floor, pulling the bar to the abdomen, aiming for the navel. The back should stay at a slight angle, the shoulders higher than the hips rather than flat-backed. Pull the elbows as high as possible while keeping the back from rounding and the body steady. If you cannot pull to the body, lower the amount of weight. Change the grip for the next set and again perform 11 repetitions, adding weight if you get all 11, dropping weight if you don't. Perform a total of 4 sets, two grips of each, of 11 reps per set.

THE SQUAT - LEGS

This is the number one lower body exercise. It is not dangerous or detrimental in any way when done correctly. It is performed by every athlete in every sport, male and female, from high school athletics, to college and semi-professional sports and throughout the professional ranks.

The squat works the hips, the gluteus, the quadriceps, the hamstrings, the calves, the ankles and the stabilizers in the stomach and lower back by having the weight balanced on the shoulders. It is the number one movement for adding speed because the force of gravity against the ground is countered by the amount of weight sustained over the shoulders, building explosive power on the running plane.

This is easy to learn, either on a Smith machine or with a barbell. But the best initial practice is with no bar at all, squatting as low as possible with the back held straight, the shoulders high, the gaze slightly upward, the toes pointing forward, the heels on the ground throughout the movement and the thighs lowered to parallel.

Place the arms out in front for counter-balance, parallel to the floor. After this warm-up set of 11 repetitions, progress to a barbell inside a squat rack and do a light set with the matching form of the weightless set. Keep strict form, always going slow enough to maintain control and posture. Then perform 4 sets of 11 repetitions, adding weight if you get all 11, dropping weight if you don't.

Avoid adding too much weight too soon, so as to not compromise form. It is imperative to do full repetitions to get the full benefit of the exercise, contrary to what you may witness by some athletes exercising their egos with wide-stance-mini-reps, exploding faces and more support straps than a truck carrying rolled steel. Slow, controlled, steady, identical repetitions allow the body to grow at its natural rate while enlisting the supporting musculatures and tendons to also get stronger.

THE MILITARY PRESS - SHOULDERS

This works the whole upper body region from the mid-chest upward.   When done correctly, as explained, it works the anterior, posterior and medial heads of the deltoids, as well as the stabilizers in the hips and lower back, with slight stimulation to the triceps, back and chest. The shoulders do not require lifting much weight due to their physically small size and three divisions. It is more beneficial, and safer for the rest of the body, to push steadily through the movement and hold at the top. This helps bring out the medial tie-ins to the triceps and biceps and aids stability in the lower back. The Military Press is the singular, best shoulder exercise.

Grasp a barbell outside shoulder width. Bring it to rest across the collarbone, either by lifting it there from the floor, or from a press rack. Place the feet shoulder width apart, the lower back and abs held tight. Press the bar overhead, holding the extended position for a two count, keeping the core fully engaged throughout the repetitions. If you are using a barbell rack, bring the bar back to the collarbone before walking forward to rest it in the upright pegs. Perform 4 sets of 11 repetitions, adding weight if you get all 11, dropping weight if you don't.

The Military Press has many variations, from the Clean to the Push-press, but this Basic movement is the foundation on which the others must be built. Rarely are you called upon to put that much weight over your head on a given day, but once shoulder strength is balanced to leg and torso strength, explosive power throughout the body is enhanced and available when called upon.

THE BARBELL CURL - BICEPS

This exercise has many variations. The barbell curl is the most widely used and still one of the most effective. The bicep is used often in many varied daily activities as well as sports. Every thing you lift and bring toward you engages the biceps muscles. This exercise aids in grip and pulling strength, and overall arm strength. It also adds a visually pleasing curve to the arms.

Grasp a barbell with the palms up, from where the hands hang straight down from the shoulders. This is the mechanically proper grip. Keep the thumbs under the bar, in a "monkey grip" which allows full development to the lower-outer portion of the biceps. The core should stay engaged for stability; drop the shoulders and shoulder blades down and back so you retain a posture of rigid straightness, rather than leaning forward toward the bar. Using just the biceps and forearms, curl the bar up to the neck, keeping the wrists straight, and the chin parallel to the floor. Add a good contraction at the top of each repetition and finish with a slow, controlled descent. Perform 4 sets of 11 repetitions, adding weight if you get all 11, dropping weight if you don't.

THE CALF RAISE - CALVES

The calves carry you every step of every day. You lift your entire body weight with one leg, each step, everywhere. They take much stimulation and can endure much work, so do not be afraid to keep the repetitions and the weight high on this exercise.

Many calf machines of varying angles and intensities are available in most gyms, but the simplest is a 4 – 6 inch step and a pair of dumbbells. This style will incorporate balance as well as foot strength and flexibility.

Stand on a step or a short ledge with the feet supported only by the toes, back to the ball of the foot, across the widest portion of the feet. Stretch the heels toward the floor, (holding on to a light bar for initial balance, but get rid of it as soon as possible), then pushing up to raise the body up as high as you can onto your toes. Do an initial set of 22 repetitions without weight, then grasp a pair of dumbbells in each hand and do 4 more sets of 22 repetitions. The weight should be enough to challenge the calves, but not too much to make the upper body struggle to hold them.

THE WRIST CURL - FOREARMS

This is another often overlooked muscle group which many athletes, male and female, avoid training. Indirectly, many other exercises utilize them, but by avoiding direct stimulation of the wrists and forearms, they become the weak link in grip strength, arm fatigue and manipulation of the upper arm in any sports requiring ballistic power and endurance.

Grasp a barbell with an underhand grip, thumbs under the bar. Then, resting the forearms on a weight bench for support, in a crouch facing the foot of the bench, with the arms locked between the legs, let the hands dangle off the edge of the bench while holding the barbell. Squeeze the bar up with just the forearms and wrists. Lower the bar to a full extension but do not let the bar roll down to the fingertips, simply flex the hands upward and down, performing 22 repetitions for a total of 4 sets. The weight used is not as crucial as the form. Do not try this with more weight than you can lift for all 22 repetitions. Instead, get as much flexibility from the wrists in a full range of motion from top to bottom for the entire movement.

THE BARBELL SHRUG - NECK/TRAPEZIUS

This exercise, like the Row for the Back, should be done with two different grips to stimulate both the front face and rear tie-ins of the muscles. The small muscles that support the head, neck and posture need the strength and stimulation this exercise offers. The added blood flow helps alleviate headaches, neck aches and counters "desk posture" by bringing the shoulders up and back; as well as opening the collarbones and strengthening the muscles of the "jowls".

Grasp a barbell behind the body, with the fingers pointed backward, and "shrug" the bar upward in a straight line as if trying to touch the ears with the shoulders. This grip stimulates the trapezius and rhomboids of the upper back and shoulders. Keep the chin parallel to the floor as you stretch up and down in the first set of 11 shrugs. Rest. Resume. Since the rhomboids, trapezius and rear deltoids are on the back of the body, it makes sense to train these muscles from this angle. Too many athletes face the bar and use too much weight, causing the shoulders to slump further forward instead of rolling them up and back as the next grip specifies. The greater stimulus comes from having the back to the bar, while lifting up and away from the

S *PORT*

You must determine the type of movement the sport requires. Is it short bursts of speed in 10 yards or less? Are you involved in long, sustained runs? Is no running required? Do you jump? How much strength do you need to move apparatus, people, your body? How long a duration do you have to keep moving? These and other considerations will greatly determine the type of Specific Training one must do.

A hockey player must train for speed in both short and middle distance sprints. He must train for lateral movement. He must train for quick stops with directional change; he must train for the strength of having to move other people traveling both in the same and opposite directions; train for agility in foot speed and hand-eye coordination using his arms which also stop the puck to pass or change the direction of it. With so many facets involved in the sport, it's best to train in as many disciplines as possible, as well as repeatedly performing the basic skills necessary to participate.

Training for baseball would require a whole other set of performance criteria. Every sport must be examined on as many levels as possible to determine the overall design of a program.

When that is determined, one takes the specifics and breaks them down into priorities to ensure that the weakest links get the first attention when brain power and energy are at their highest, at the beginning of the workout. This is where most athletes fail. They do what they're comfortable with, either in the gym or weight room or on the field, and save little time or energy for their weakest links, often running out of time and skipping the most necessary training rather than training the weakness to make that link stronger.

In sports where great force need be used with spontaneity and fluidity and often, great accuracy, one must train the body for ballistic movement. Plyometrics training answers explosive ability. Rehearsal/mimicry answers accuracy.

Racket sports, baseball, basketball, hockey, lacrosse, soccer, football and many more sports require the body to use its force in one direction, stop an object and fire it back in the opposite direction. This is a great strain on the body, especially when done repetitively.

SPECIFIC BASICS

By narrowing down the movements to allow the required strength and corresponding growth to occur takes a number of variables that make specific movements crucial to getting the body to respond as desired. Changing the hand grip, the angle of the bench, the type of bar, the height of the machine, the weight, the reps scheme, the order of exercises, the gravity of the movement all add to the stress put on the muscle and the resulting effect created by that type of exercise. Specificity in exercise takes attention, patience, control, experimentation, research, feedback and open-mindedness. Some people drink milk and some drink honey before a race. What makes each work is the belief coming from the athlete that this way, is his way, which he's learned from trial and accomplishment. What the mind believes, the body achieves. It is not skepticism nor superstition, but based on belief and application over various trials and the knowledge that comes from feeling your way through certain exercises, making that mind/body connection that happens on the athletic level when we're open to it and when conscious attention is paid to cultivating its availability for future performances.

The order of weight training should always be:

WARM UP – full movements, light repetitions, complete range of motion, high repetitions.

COMPOUND MOVEMENTS FIRST – Compound movements involve two or more joints; wrist, elbow and shoulder; ankle, knee, and hip. These are primarily the movements where you can use the most weight and hit the largest concentration of muscle fibers. These include: the bench press, the military press and the clean for upper body; and the stiff-legged deadlift, leg press and squat for the lower body.

ISOLATED, CONCENTRATED MOVEMENTS LAST – These are the refining movements like the concentration curl for the biceps, the triceps pushdown, the leg extension and the flye. During these movements, the fewer the moving joints, the more concentrated the movement.

ISOMETRIC OR FREEHAND MOVEMENTS – These can either be used as a warm up or cool down. Pull ups, push-ups, lunges, sit-ups, and dips are great moves to warm up in a full range of motion or to squeeze the last bit of energy out of the end of a workout.

"We only learn our limits by going beyond them. "

8

<u>FEEDBACK</u>

"Whosoever Knows Others Is Clever

Whosoever Knows Himself Is Wise.

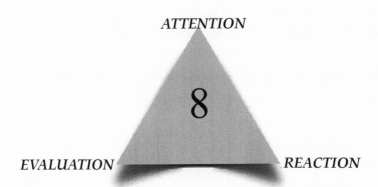

FEEDBACK

To know an opponent is often an exercise in futility. You can watch past performances, read statistics, watch them train in the gym or on the field, but you will never know all they have to offer. There will be that unknown piece of their makeup that can't be visibly seen or measured by observation. You can't gauge their passion, drive, desire or preparations. As hard as you may try to learn about an opponent, there will be a limit and a certain degree of mystery.

The same holds true for that person knowing you. There is a depth to each one of us that can only be called upon from our own minds. There are resources within us that we cannot explain how they're summoned. Oftentimes we surprise ourselves with our performances.

To know a teammate in terms of trusting what they'll deliver in speed, talent or assistance is good to speculate upon, but to really know their capabilities is immeasurable. To "know others is clever" and as much as can be found in the efforts to study them is a valuable asset to any competitive training program. But time better spent is in learning about ourselves through testing, feedback, evaluation and retesting.

The key in studying feedback is the "wisdom" found in "knowing oneself". "Whosoever knows himself is wise" means you've paid enough attention to the aspects and variations in your own training to know your capabilities under various circumstances. Knowing yourself through continuous trial and effort brings a sense of confidence to the field that regular practice alone cannot. By knowing the depth and intensity of your own training brings courage in attitude and assuredness to performance.

Simply charting your progress against the goals you've set is feedback. Recording what you plan to do and then writing what you've accomplished is the reality check that makes you above average. By seeing in black and white, where you started, where you're at, and where you're headed has a compounding effect that leads to positive approaches for future endeavors. When you see that you could only do 2 push-ups or pull-ups when you began, and now record sets of 11, 22, or more is a stimulus to reach higher yet.

WHAT IS FEEDBACK?

The feedback of a workout regimen involves many aspects to consider. One must know why each move benefits the body, how much to do, when to back off, how to cycle the training, what foods to eat and an ongoing list of checks and balances to evaluate how well the approach is working. By using, utilizing and applying this feedback on an ongoing basis, the athlete learns about himself and the wisdom becomes his own.

By observing these same aspects of role models to emulate performance, makes the athlete clever in recognizing what can be borrowed and what should be left alone. We learn not only by doing, but also by observing. If someone is where you want to be, you model them until you know what it takes to be in that position, then, you pass them. When you are humble enough to respect your own weaknesses, you begin to know how to work with them to delete them.

Feedback is essential because it helps to gauge our progress within a given exercise. Does your back hurt? Are you feeling the movement more in the shoulders than the pectorals? Are you having more pains since beginning workouts? What are you doing wrong? Weight lifting programs are supposed to make you stronger, feel better, shape faster, and perform longer at higher intensities. If these things aren't happening, then you must ask, "why?" That is feedback.

Feedback is a measurement. It could be as vague as how you feel, or as specific as a millisecond of time. It is a way to gauge progress or lack of it. Feedback is another way of paying attention to how your body is performing. It can be witnessed by outside observers, but it is best evaluated by your own personal measurement. Feedback builds with Specifics and holds you accountable for your own progress.

THIS IS ONLY A TEST

The following tests and charts are standard ways to test strength and flexibility with common measurements that anyone can have access to. It is important to try as many of these as possible, just to get a baseline measurement for where you stand. A common cycle is to do the test at the beginning of a new regimen, then again after a 6-week cycle to gauge improvements. Tests can be done more often, but should at least minimally be performed every month, or each time a training style is changed or new exercises incorporated.

We will often weigh ourselves every day and sometimes more when on a new diet, but never take into account if the other aspects of our health are helping in a measurable way. Knowing how to test speed, strength and flexibility are essential to our fitness ability. Do not avoid knowing these crucial factors and working to improve them.

FIVE FACTORS DETERMINE FITNESS LEVEL

1. Body Composition - these cannot be changed
   A. Endomorph – slim frame, narrow joints, small ankles and wrists
   B. Ectomorph – thick frame, heavy joints, ankles and wrists
   C. Mesomorph – athletic frame, well-proportioned, not too thick or thin

2. <u>Diet</u> – this can definitely be changed
   A. high fats and / or carbohydrates, little protein
   B. high proteins, lean meats, little carbohydrate
   C. balance of protein, carbohydrates and fats
3. <u>Aerobic/ Cardiovascular Conditioning</u> – essential to every athlete
   A. no conditioning
   B. overly conditioned aerobically, but little strength or flexibility
   C. balance of cardiovascular, strength and flexibility training
4. <u>Strength</u> – can and must be improved and sustained
   A. overly musclebound, but disproportionate amidst muscle groups
   B. weak muscle tone and little bodyweight strength
   C. muscle tone in proportion to whole body with minimal weaknesses
5. <u>Flexibility</u> – can and must be improved and sustained
   A. a rubberband with eyeballs
   B. so tight one can't reach up, down or across the body comfortably
   C. good range across the shoulders, lower back, hamstrings and overhead

The only factor that cannot be changed in this list are the body type you are born with. The rest of the spectrum can be worked on, enhanced, improved and balanced. The first two choices are exaggerated examples of people who go too far in any one direction. The last examples state balance and proportion and are what every person should strive to achieve, athlete and non-athlete.

REMOVE THE NUMBERS

Too often, people are hung up in the numbers, "how much weight they'll loose, how much weight they can push, how many repetitions, how many minutes, how much longer? In just 15 minutes a day... The 10 best exercises..."

Remove all the numbers from the plates and forget the sets and reps. Numbers are only a gauge. They are simply a way of reaffirming to yourself that you're doing x amount of y and it always comes out to z; the result is in direct proportion to the effort exerted. We are not after numbers. We are after results. Once a good level of fitness is achieved, it is hard to give up, and then it becomes hard to live without, literally and figuratively. All exercise should lead you within your body, as well as show you how to transcend it. When you learn to begin paying close attention to the movement, the numbers will stop mattering

Use numbers like a mantra to get through your sets, whether they're two forced repetitions or 110 reps sets. Put intensity into every one and you'll have to do less, yet gain better results at a faster rate. If you work the mind with the muscle, the mind/body connection doubles the benefit. Numbers count in our measured, analyzed, rated, graded, judged world. But to the internal world of the true athlete, the reward is the preparation, the performance and the victory of overcoming obstacles both personal and external.

The most important part of exercise is the "feel" you're getting from it. Feedback simply means listening to our bodies. You feel "the pump..." "the burn..." "if you feel faint or dizzy, step off the machine..." Once we listen to our bodies and how they're responding to a workout, we'll begin to get more from our workouts.

When we stop listening to our bodies, it's like the analogy of turning up our car radio when a sound we don't want to hear presents itself. We shut off the pain, we medicate, we deny, cheat or disregard the creaks and crackles of joints all in the name of "feeling" we are doing best for our bodies by rising above the noises they make. A shoulder injury, if not taken care of, moves to the shoulder blade area and up toward the neck, then down to the mid-back, the lower back, and eventually to the hip and down the leg. This transference of pain is simply the supporting muscles trying to alleviate the stress to the injury. But the blockage was not removed, so you're causing a log jam of blood flow and oxygen supply to the nerves and muscles. Before long, a small, workable injury becomes a detriment not only to your training, but to your normal movements and lifestyle.

Rest is just as crucial to training progress as nutrition and the training itself. Rest and reflection balance the mind and body while healing it on a more thorough level. We hit plateau's to see that our routines have become stagnant or that our bodies have switched into accommodation – the point where muscles are so accustomed to that particular movement that they respond by rote – monotonously, like bricklayers laying bricks - and they accommodate by doing what they can already do under however great a load is put upon them. Or they break down. Function often outlasts form.

F.E.E.D.B.A.C.K

F *ORMULAS* – The Karvonen and Body Mass Index for heartrate and weight.

E *SSENTIAL* – Knowing your progress through feedback inspires and reins you in.

E *VALUATE* – Pay attention to what your training is doing and how you're feeling.

D *IET* – Define what you're eating, how much, and how certain foods affect the way you   feel and perform.

B *ENEFITS* - Conscientious feedback enables continuous benefits

A *SSESS* - Basic tests to help you gauge your athletic abilities as they currently stand

C *ALCULATE* – With your starting point, you can project future goals and possibility.

K *NOWLEDGE* – After this battery of tests and trials, you'll know what needs work.

F *ORMULAS*

The two initial formulas to see where you stand and to observe fitness progress are the Karvonen formula to monitor maximum heart rate zones and the Body Mass Index (BMI) which gives a height to weight ratio as a guideline to heart health and disease.

The BMI is simply the tape-measurement around the belly button and its relationship to your height in inches. The circumference of your stomach should be half or less than your height in inches. If you are 72 inches tall, than your waist measurement should be less than 36 inches.   The following chart details the risks associated with a higher Body Mass Index.

The Karvonen Formula is a measurement of optimal heartrate training zones based on initial resting heart rates (RHR). In order to find them, you must first find your average resting heart rate, which can be measured over three consecutive mornings upon awakening. They can also be taken after remaining seated for 30 to 60 minutes, but the more accurate measure is done in the morning upon awakening. This example is based on a 35 year old person. The lower measurement is the bottom end of the training zone (65%), and the higher number represents the higher (85%), more advanced training zone. Staying within these zones provide optimum fat burning and cardiovascular benefit and can be sustained in aerobic or strength training exercise.

KARVONEN FORMULA

TRAINING HEART RATE = resting heart rate x intensity + resting heart rate

Example: 35 year old male

220 – 35 (age) =185

185 – 60 (resting heart rate) = 125

125 x 65% (low end of training zone) = 81.25 + 60

(resting heart rate) = 141.25

125 x 85% (high end of training zone) = 106.25 + 60 (RHR) =166.25 Optimal Training Heart Rate Zone for a 35 year old male w/60 (RHR) is 141 – 166 bpm

This simply means that training within these heart rate zones will garner the most fat burning and cardiovascular building results.

BODY MASS INDEX (Height to Hip ratio)

To use the table, find the appropriate height in the left-hand column. Move across the row to the given weight. The number at the top of the column is the BMI for that height and weight.

BMI (kg/m)	19	20	21	22	23	24	25	26	27	28	29	30	35	40
Height (in.)	Weight (lb.)													
58	91	96	100	105	110	115	119	124	129	134	138	143	167	191
59	94	99	104	109	114	119	124	128	133	138	143	148	173	198
60	97	102	107	112	118	123	128	133	138	143	148	153	179	204
61	100	106	111	116	122	127	132	137	143	148	153	158	185	211
62	104	109	115	120	126	131	136	142	147	153	158	164	191	218
63	107	113	118	124	130	135	141	146	152	158	163	169	197	225

64	110	116	122	128	134	140	145	151	157	163	169	174	204	232
65	114	120	126	132	138	144	150	156	162	168	174	180	210	240
66	118	124	130	136	142	148	155	161	167	173	179	186	216	247
67	121	127	134	140	146	153	159	166	172	178	185	191	223	255
68	125	131	138	144	151	158	164	171	177	184	190	197	230	262
69	128	135	142	149	155	162	169	176	182	189	196	203	236	270
70	132	139	146	153	160	167	174	181	188	195	202	207	243	278
71	136	143	150	157	165	172	179	186	193	200	208	215	250	286

72	140	147	154	162	169	177	184	191	199	206	213	221	258	294
73	144	151	159	166	174	182	189	197	204	212	219	227	265	302
74	148	155	163	171	179	186	194	202	210	218	225	233	272	311
75	152	160	168	176	184	192	200	208	216	224	232	240	279	319
76	156	164	172	180	189	197	205	213	221	230	238	246	287	328

Risk of Associated Disease According to BMI and Waist Size			
BMI		Waist less than or equal to 40 in. (men) or 35 in. (women)	Waist greater than 40 in. (men) or 35 in. (women)

18.5 or less	Underweight	--	N/A
18.5 - 24.9	Normal	--	N/A
25.0 - 29.9	Overweight	Increased	High
30.0 - 34.9	Obese	High	Very High
35.0 - 39.9	Obese	Very High	Very High
40 or greater	Extremely Obese	Extremely High	Extremely High

Based on these two formulas, you can begin with measurements to know where you stand in relation to national averages and start your program accordingly. As your weight and bodyfat decrease, and cardiovascular capacity increases, your inches lost around the belly will also decrease, thus, lowering susceptibility to many dangerous diseases. Attention to diet alone can decrease risk, as can exercise alone, but done in combination of diet and exercise, the results occur quicker and many additional benefits come from strength and aerobic training with attention to diet.

FIVE STEPS TO SUCCESS FOR GAINS IN STRENGTH, SPEED, SIZE, AGILITY

1. TEST – a number, a baseline, a checkpoint, a compass to show where you stand
2. EVALUATE – do you feel you could do better, be better, achieve better scores
3. SET GOALS – go after what you feel possible to accomplish in time and ability
4. FOLLOW PLANS FOR IMPROVEMENT – walk the walk, talk the talk
5. TEST AGAIN – honest assessment of what you've accomplished and how much you truly put in toward improvement in time, attention and tuition.

E *SSENTIAL*

Feedback is essential in order to understand you are making measurable progress through realizing what techniques, apparatus, routines, diets, weights and repertoires work best for your body type and activity level. It is essential to know your body enough to know when a certain pain is positive or negative toward your progress. It is essential to have feedback to know if you are on your way toward your projected goal, when to raise the bar and when to retreat or regroup toward another approach.

Essential feedback is something as easy as looking in the mirror and seeing less of the belly sticking over the beltline, more shape or tone to the shoulders and arms, a tighter jawline, a more-pronounced chin. All these little nuances add positively to the fire that keeps you going, knowing that this exercise works, with evident, measurable benefits you can actually see on a daily basis. It is absolutely essential to keep some type of feedback *'feeding back"* to your mind and instilling that what you're doing is not in vain, whether it be a positive blood test result, better sleep and sex, or the way an old suit fits.

It is not essential to memorize and compartmentalize any series of foods or routines or measurements that are some arbitrary ideal you must meet. It is only necessary to pay attention through how you look and feel to recognize your efforts.

E *VALUATE*

You must gather enough information over a long enough period of time with the same set of parameters to be able to evaluate if this process is working for you. As you learn your feedback cycle you must use a consistent set of criteria to honestly assess if this combination is giving you the best results. Sometimes changing exercise order, or doing cardio training before strength training or vice versa, will give different benefits that only are evidenced when evaluating the program as a whole. Evaluation is a judgment to prove that $x + y = z$, and if it doesn't, where does it fail and where can it be improved?

To evaluate your feedback it is best to use concrete numbers and results. Where it's ok to have a subjective opinion to realize that feedback is essential, that it "looks" like you're making progress; with evaluation you have concrete, measurable numbers to say, "I did 33 minutes of cardio for 5 days in a row and lost 2.2 pounds." or, "I could only do 2 sets of 5 pushups two weeks ago and now I do 3 sets of 11," you're evaluating with proven facts that following this regimen produces this result. And it also works in finding that a certain routine produces no measurable result and you then reevaluate the routine to incorporate the things that will garner results. You add value to feedback.

D *IET*

How does diet refer to feedback? How do your pants fit? Diet is crucial toward feedback on any training regimen and the more attention paid to it, the faster and better the results. High endurance athletes need carbohydrates, bodybuilders and strength athletes need protein, and we all need fats. It all comes down to the amounts, types and timing of the correct foods that determine results. Some people must eat as soon as they wake up. Some can wait until 11 or 12 before they feel the need to have a meal. Some say they do not need to eat more than toast and coffee to start their day.

This is where I disagree. The first meal should be eaten within an hour after awakening and should consist of protein, fats and carbohydrates. There are so many recipes to be made with this balance of nutrients, but eating on a regular basis, with adequate portions and more protein than carbohydrates will benefit the athlete and non-athlete equally.

If you choose to train first thing in the morning, than a different combinations of foods are necessary with the balance going toward carbohydrates, but the higher protein still applies. The crucial factor is getting good fuel into your body as soon as possible to alleviate the possibility of grazing the wrong things that first come into sight at work or when rushing everyone else out the door and 'picking' at the remains. An apple for the drive is better than a bagel. Add some walnuts and some orange or grapefruit juice and you've made a permissible choice. But this is only an occasional indulgence and should not be the norm for a balanced breakfast.

All meals should include this balance of protein, carbohydrates and fats. The best choice for lunch is a Waldorf or "Wow" salad. A "wow" salad is one that when it arrives at your table, you're inclined to say, "wow!" It should include tuna, salmon or chicken and a wide array of vegetables in addition to nuts, apples, a few dried fruits and a minimum of dressing, but preferably lemon juice or oil and vinegar. The more varied the types of vegetables, from peppers to cabbages and radishes, the more beneficial the salad will be for your digestive and respiratory systems. The bulk will keep you full longer and aid in elimination later.

For dinner, choices should be lighter than lunch. It should be consumed before 7 p.m. and eaten slowly, over the course of at least 30 minutes. Desert should be an occasional indulgence and used as a reward rather than a necessary end to the meal. Fresh, raw fruit is advisable any time but avoid "no or low-fat" toppings. Just eat more fruit. Breads and pastas should also be treated like "treats" rather than staples. The only staple they provide is when they do the gastric bypass and staple your stomach closed! Use food to see how you feel during exercise and events and the feedback you get from your performance will help determine optimal amounts and types for your training.

B *ENEFITS*

The benefits of feedback are compounded by the length of time you watch them. Every single area of your fitness can be improved through feedback and the resulting action you take to steer them toward your goals. The benefits include making greater progress in less amount of time and energy, alleviating weaknesses, enhancing your physique, overall health and knowing when any part of it is off so it can be easily corrected.

One of the most valuable benefits to paying attention to feedback is the ability to trust your body in what it's saying to you when you're injured, tired or sore. If you're aware an exercise will leave the certain soreness you've come to expect from it, you'll know whether to add that extra day of basketball in after a leg session if you're privy to the amount of soreness it will leave you with. The benefit of knowing your body will come in handy when a cold comes on, when a backache persists, when cramps are evident and you don't know whether or not you should work around them. By knowing yourself through feedback, these questions will be easily answered second-naturedly.

A *SSESS*

FOUR SIMPLE TESTS TO ASSESS FITNESS LEVELS

TEST	*EXPECTED RESULT*
1.5 mile running endurance test	less than 18 minutes
Push – up test	33 in 1 minute min.

Sit-ups in crunch position

                        44 in 1 minute min.

Flexibility – reach between legs in seated position on
floor   19 inches forward

A SECOND SIMPLE FLEXIBILITY TEST FOR BACK AND HAMSTRINGS

Hold a broomstick overhead in front of a full-length mirror. Squat down as far as possible, butt to heels, and observe:

- Heels come up – tight Achilles tendons; lean forward on front leg and stretch inner thigh
- Body not straight – tight hip flexors and lower back; kneel with leg at 90°, stretch hip flexors by pulling gently on the foot of bent knee on the floor
- Unlocked elbows/ head down – chest and shoulders too tight; place arm against stationary object, arm bent at 90° to gently stretch shoulders and chest

VERTICAL JUMP TEST

Stand tall and reach to the highest mark on the wall. Jump up and mark highest touch:

AGE (yrs.)	20-29	30-39	40-49	50-59
HEIGHT OF JUMP FROM INITIAL STANDING MARK				
Superior	26.5+	25+	22+	21+
Excellent	24-26	22.5-24	19-22	17-21
Good	21.5-23	20-22	17-18.5	15-16.5
Poor	17.5-19.5	16.5-18	14-15	12-13

SPEED PERFORMANCE TESTS

Attempt each one of these dashes with someone standing by to time you. These sprints are relative to the athlete's gender, age, weight, condition and training level. This will give you a starting point to see where initial speed is, and periodic testing will reveal which distances and types best suit your speed style. It is not necessary to test all distances in one day, but if you do, go longest to shortest distance when energy and interest are at their highest. Perform on a high school or college marked track.

440 yard dash – *a helper with a stopwatch is the best way to get accurate readings*

300 yard shuttle run – mark 25 yards and make 12 total passes, approx. 11 secs. each

220 yard dash – one half time around the track

100 yard dash – the length of a football field, as marked

50 yard dash – half the length of a football field
40 yard dash – the baseline measurement for speed on
most athletic teams
20 yard dash – test for initial speed

STRENGTH TESTS

These are all very subjective and relative to the athlete's gender, age, weight, condition and training level. Each movement should be tested with light enough weight to ensure proper form and range of motion over a minimum of 4 repetitions.

After a warm – up set with a manageable weight, proceed to second set at 85% maximum capability for 3-4 repetitions, then 3rd and 4th sets with a spotter to attempt two repetitions with perfect form. This will give you a baseline of your strength. The test sets should be of maximum effort. A warm-up set of 15-20 repetitions should be done prior to each attempted movement unless noted.

Squat –Warm-up, a set of 3-4 repetitions at 85%
maximum, 2 attempts at 1 Rep Max
Bench Press - Warm-up, a set of 3-4 repetitions at
85% maximum, 2 attempts at 1 RM
Bent Over Row - Warm-up, a set of 3-4
repetitions at 85% maximum, 2 attempts at 1 RM

Barbell Curl - Warm-up, a set of 3-4 repetitions at 85% maximum, 2 attempts at 1 RM
Military Press - Warm-up, a set of 3-4 repetitions at 85% maximum, 2 attempts at 1 RM
Pull-ups – You should be warmed up, 2 attempts at maximum number of full repetitions
Dips - You should be warmed up, 2 attempts at maximum number of full repetitions

This initial assessment must be taken with an objective point of view. If you had never attempted some of these activities or tests prior to this outing, you should not expect too high of results. If you had taken these types of tests before, many years ago, than it's an eye-opening experience that should also be taken with a grain of salt for the fact that the condition your body is presently in, compared to where you were on prior testing, is a different body entirely. The best assessment comes in doing these tests periodically from this point forward to see your capability for improvement. Write goals based on these numbers and you have a beginning point to focus your work upon.

C ALCULATE

Let the formulas, the tests and the baselines be your guide to future accomplishments. Calculate how far off you are from your ideal Body Mass Index, your flexibility and your ideal strength. Know your heart rate and its ideal low and high numbers. Factor your calories consumed against your calories expended and calculate how long it will take to reach your ideal weight or fitness level.

This feedback is essential to gauge where you've come from and where you're going to. Watch attentively for a month how your times in the sprint runs improve and how the starting weights and maximum weights in your strength lifts add up to a new and improved you. Chart your progress in a notebook that only contains your workouts and be amazed years later when you glance back through it at how capable you are. By realizing through feedback that progress comes in small increments as well as giant leaps, you will be more prone to set higher and harder goals for your future progress.

K NOWLEDGE

Knowledge is power. By using this Simple Structured Training System to gauge your physicality, you will have in place a knowledge base that is as vital as any stock portfolio, physician's folder, or reference manual which you can view as your blueprint for fitness, and the developing course you've taken toward improvement. Many people make the mistake of hit and missing their way toward fitness, based on advice or attempts at something seen in magazines rather than first-hand accounts of what got you to great shape. When you have the breadth of knowledge that these feedback tests offer, you have a bonafide plan that led you step by step from a place of a uncertain condition to a place of greater conditioning. Armed with these facts, you have something to substantiate when your will or mind come up weak, that "yes, something better is possible."

"Whatever you are, be a good one."

9

<u>SPORTS</u>

"Whosoever Conquers Others Has Force.

Whosoever Conquers Himself Is Strong."

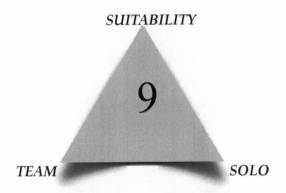

SUITABILITY

9

TEAM   SOLO

ACQUIRING FORCE AND STRENGTH

"Whosoever conquers others" in sport, is the definition of competition. To rise victorious in games of skill, precision, timing and split-second decisions are what make up a great part of our world culture. It is war without death, achieving in the spirit of sportsmanship by holding your foe in gratitude and mutual admiration when the battle is done. Sports performance hinges on the training done off the field and the ability of the athlete to bring that training to the game. It means possessing the energy, endurance and strength required for extended durations of concentrated effort, determination and focus. This is the acquisition and ownership of "force."

To conquer with force is to out-distance, out-think, out-train, and out-play your opponents with a tenacity that wears them down while winding you up. "Whosoever conquers others has force" means that it is something you come to the table with, you don't find it on the field or on the way to the game. You arrive with the force necessary to get the job done. "Whosoever... HAS." That force may come in adrenaline, belief, vindictiveness or pure brute strength, but the force that wins the contest is an intrinsic component established with practice and preparedness as physical as any piece of equipment, as obvious as a helmet, as recognizable as the number on your back. To have force is to consistently demonstrate the mind/body/spirit resources the event requires.

"Conquers himself," means knowing the strengths, weaknesses and idiosyncrasies that make you unique. To conquer yourself is to take that leap into the ultimate plane where you know and are capable of your job and perform it with a flow to make it appear effortless. Conquering yourself is taking any weaknesses and squeezing them out of your body and mind so only strength survives. As an athlete in any sport, even for everyday fitness, you must conquer the mental demons that plague acceptance on so many levels. Past performance does not equal future performance. If you recognize a failure from the past and then work optimistically to build both mental and physical strength to avoid that happening again, you've squeezed out a weakness and gained positive programming to realize what's possible in future endeavors.

To conquer oneself is to be strong in every aspect of discipline, from the mental to the physical to the spiritual, and smart enough to recognize and admit when one is on the way to breaking down. This preserves strength. Strength holds one end of the body to the other, the mind to the feet, the heart to the hands. In all sports you must have a strong determination, a strong physicality, and an inner strength that comes as confidence in knowing your preparations were thorough and complete. "Whosoever conquers himself" has already won over the greatest opponent.

MENTAL/ PHYSICAL/ SPIRITUAL

Believing, visualizing, adopting a positive attitude and creating a beneficial scenario to foster an ideal environment are the mental aspects. If it turns out your belief doesn't bear fruit, you must reevaluate your route, your approach and your capabilities. By thinking of how long you have before a specific target date, and by breaking the training into achievable increments, keeps your training in perspective and allows more force or more rest as needed.

Concentration and focus must be strengthened like any other characteristic and not just by repeatedly performing the necessary actions. The concentration necessary in an optimal golf swing can be learned in the guided, centering practices of Pilates sessions in addition to repeated drives. Training outside of your sport is imperative to bringing the optimum benefits from varied disciplines to the whole gamut that is your game.

The physical lies in proper rest, nutrition, recuperation and execution of movements in practice. By compensating with adjustments for energy levels and the reality of variables not written into the regiment, the tone is set for the injury-free training found in focused attention.　Every aspect you incorporate into your physical make-up in training – strength, flexibility, balance – is called upon on the playing field at the most unexpected moments.　A well-trained body doesn't get simple injuries while walking out to the field or warming up.　Injuries come from poor preparation, inattention, physical weakness, or freak accidents when more force is exerted on appendages and joints than they are capable of withstanding. To the opposite effect, if the physical is over-trained, it can also lead to accidents, mistakes or injuries through overzealousness and loss of control, hindering not only the athlete but also jeopardizing the whole team.

The spiritual contains all the other aspects within it. The spiritual is the underlying awareness as all this preparedness unfolds for you. You know when you're treating your body good. You also know if you're abusing it. So you should learn how to use it in a positive fashion so it continues to grow, adapt and react naturally. Spirit may show up as intuition, as gut-reaction, and as a sixth-sense that will be listened to only if the awareness of it is trained along with the physical aspects.

Knowing yourself, your limits, your capabilities and knowing when to push the boundaries are evident in spirit.　Sometimes spirit itself takes over and raises the whole level of performance to something magical that will forever be a barometer for future measurement. It's as important to train the spirit to avoid its breakdown, as it is any other part of preparation.

Spirit encompasses attitude, beliefs and physical preparations. Spirit lifts you when you're down and sustains you when you must go on. Spirit is exhibited when the miraculous play happens out of thin air. It is the thread that weaves each aspect to the other in an impenetrable, invisible bond.

SUITABILITY

You must find the sport that suits you. Not all sports are one-size fits all. That's why jockeys are jockeys, sumo wrestlers are sumo wrestlers and basketball players are basketball players. Some sports suit body styles and capabilities better than others and the sooner you can find the best fit, the better off you are; but on the way there, try as many sports, pastimes and activities as accessibility allows.

All sports require fluid movement, timing and concentration. Some sports require hitting objects, some throwing, some kicking and some, fighting. The way you train for each of these should be as individual as the sport. If you don't like running long distances, cannot swim and don't own a bicycle, don't choose to be a triathlete.

In relation to your sport, is most of the movement forward? Lateral? Vertical? Does it require power, finesse, speed, or endurance? How big is the field? What are the conditions you play under - sun, mud? The more you can answer these questions and prepare in every way for whatever combination of energies are required, the more successful you will be at taking the body you have and applying it to the sport of choice. Suitability is a uniform for the body's abilities, exhibited best when wearing well your God-given attributes.

SOLO

An athlete like Olympic swimmer Michael Phelps doesn't think of how he's going to perform, he simply performs his best and practices hard, always, until it's so natural that he does it effortlessly. He is already there, doing what he does as if there were no other way. He knows his capabilities, pushes beyond them every single stroke, and answers only to his own voice. Coaches and supporters and teammates may be helping him along, but it's he, himself, whose mind has decided that nothing will stand in his way. His abilities will be fully utilized without compromise. His is an example of taking a solo sport and mastering every aspect of it, then continually working to improve his capabilities until he is untouchable in his sport.

There are examples of these single standout performers in many team sports. That's why we have superstars. But what got them there was there own inner drive which propelled them ahead of so many others in the same positions, on the same fields. What makes them "super" is the ability to bring superior performances repeatedly, often surpassing past accomplishments.

The mental aspect of solo sports athletes is perhaps the most crucial to develop. Their reliance is within. The most successful bodybuilders, golfers, swimmers, boxers, decathletes, cyclists and others each have to have a mental strength that oversees every part of training that supercedes outside influence and distraction. Listen intuitively if that is your chosen calling. And remember, there's always someone or something to compete against, even if it's a mountain of ice.

The solo athlete is sometime called on for teamwork, as in a relay race. He does his part to the best of his abilities but cannot bear the performance of the person he hands the baton off to. He can inspire with ignited passion, raise the level of team play in leading by example, but he can't perform the leg of the race for that next person.

TEAMS

You are on a field to play a game. You are going there to do a job better than your opponent, but never forget that he is also your co-worker. Without him, you would not have a job. Show up prepared to do a better job than anyone else.

In team play, the key word is "sharing." You share responsibilities, you share information, you share duties and you share the glory and the tears. Teamwork leads to integrity and respect, from both the self and those you participate with in the game.

It is important in team sports to practice, rehearse, train and relax with teammates because that is what helps you find out how the other person ticks. You learn their strengths and weaknesses and ways of thinking when approaching problems. You learn timing and philosophy and traded tips which help both of you to bring a higher level of play to the field. You learn human nature, and you learn that it's not entirely about you, and in order for you to do your best job, you have to help your teammate to become the best they can be.

Training for team sports requires a different approach than solo sports. Like a musician in a band or an actor in a movie, the athlete's moves must be practiced with everyone knowing their particular cue, and how one scene connects to the last and the next in a forward flowing line of action that leads to an expected outcome.

These patterns must be ingrained and known by rote in order for them to ring true each time, striking the right chord and progression of performance signposts so that everyone recognizes they are moving down the field, court, rink or track in a symphony of timing, precision, fusion and synchronicity toward a common, shared goal. Knowing what to expect from a teammate and their capabilities leans more toward improvisational acting or jazz than strict theatrics. But this room for the unexpected is built right into the practice session and therefore also seems rehearsed when the occasion to rise above normalcy is required.

S.P.O.R.T.S.

S *ELF-SUFFICIENCY* – Know what works together for your best, repeated performances.

P *OSITION* – Know what part of the event hinges on your abilities.

O *PTIMAL* – Get the greatest results with the least effort through attentive focus.

R *EQUIREMENTS* – Take into account all that's necessary for safe, continual participation.

T *IME* – Be productive and in tune with time, on and off the field.

S *TRENGTH* – Build every aspect of strength to delete all possible weaknesses.

S *ELF-SUFFICIENCY*

Self-sufficiency is when the results of the collective effort are greater than any singular part. This pertains to the other people on your team utilizing their energies toward a collective goal, if it is a team sport you pursue. In individual sports, it involves making the components of your body and training come together to perform to the best conclusion in the chosen event.

Everything must work together in the most efficient, safest, most powerful way on every level of play. The only way to force self-sufficiency to work is by preparedness. This comes more to those in individual sports, where accountability is necessary only for the self; but as a team player, when you do your part in the operation, you add the element of synchronistic unfolding when play flows your way.

An individual must train all aspects of physique and performance when the sport requires you to rely on yourself, as in triathlons or skiing, surfing or boxing. Self-sufficiency happens because training, nutrition and preparation are equally balanced and readily available when called to action.

A team player must train all aspects of the self, in addition to practicing team-timing, flow, patterned plays and tempo as learned only by working with others who contribute to a synchronistic whole as a team. The self is responsible for the role it plays in the whole enterprise. So to create self-sufficiency in both team and individual sports, note that the chain is only as strong as its weakest link.

P *OSITION*

The hockey goalie trains different than the forward or the defensemen. The basketball center trains different than the forward and the guard; the baseball catcher different than the pitcher, outfielder or infielder.

Each position on a team has a different set of parameters of which he is responsible. In volleyball, each player must know all the positions from serving to set up to spike. Examining the position on both the field and within the team gives the athlete the best perspective of his approach to training. An equestrian must ride the horse differently than the polo player, and different yet from the racer. Each person enhances his training by first realizing their position in the whole of the big picture.

Like any other aspect, you have the greatest chance of success by obtaining a versatile approach to every sport in general and your position in particular. The constant running in basketball or soccer are helped more from sprint drills than long distance mileage. The throwing and swinging found in baseball, golf or tennis benefit not from just repeated strokes, but from centering, grounding, and core work. A pole vaulter's strength must be trained in equal measure to speed, timing and explosive plyometric power. Too often an athlete looks at the one crucial moment of needed performance and overlooks the total involvement over the duration of the game.

Do you move small or large objects over various distances quickly and accurately? Do you have to outrun others while holding or controlling an object? Figure out your position and just as importantly, how all the other positions affect yours.

O *PTIMAL*

Optimizing performance and preparation requires examining the most minute, idiosyncratic aspects that the next person may not think of to garner that little edge over the competition. It's the drag of the swimsuit material against the water, or the difference between a shaved body and the resistance it causes if it's not clean-shaven in swimming or cycling.

It means giving the body adequate rest, nutrition, focus and visualization to see into the impossible. It is creating a mental, physical and spiritual environment of great promise so the resulting reaction will be natural and free-flowing. It means being ready for the gym or the game by having clothes, food, frame-of-mind and energy available to get the most out of it and not just to go through the motions. Optimal means "best possible," and that's the least you can expect.

In order to foster the optimal environment for sports you should look through the whole spectrum of all that's involved, from the best time to train, to the amount of sleep required. Not everyone needs to examine every gram of food intake, but if protein synthesis is a crucial factor as in bodybuilding, it's to your advantage to obtain and take in as many positive nutrients as a contest body requires. For the everyday athlete, if cover-model musculature is the condition desired, than the optimal route is to learn exactly what will get you there and then follow through by applying proper nutrition and training principles.

You cannot create optimal conditions dependent on weather or, like a surfer, waves. But you can prepare your body for adverse conditions and train during less-than-optimal days. So then when the days are optimal, your body will be ready for better results too. To constantly wait for optimal conditions is a lesson in futility. But to make the most of what you're given and optimizing that time with the most desirable expectations will lift training to "fun," with you in control and positive results and satisfying accomplishments even in practice.

R EQUIREMENTS

The list of requirements for a sport are more than equipment and clothing. If you practice yoga, you would have different requirements than for hockey practice or a softball game. In addition to equipment and clothing, that requirement would be attitude. If you think the training is an unnecessary waste of time; if you think preparing food or workout schedules is too much to consider; if you think you're not good enough, not ready or just not going to win or even stand a chance, then what are your chances if you begin with an attitude like this?

You are required from the outset to face every physical challenge, big or small, with the attitude that you will conquer it. Every one, every time. The professional athlete must be just as mentally optimistic that he will win the Superbowl, as the 300 pound person must be determined to lose 10 pounds per week.

You must also consider aptitude. Are you sure you're the candidate for that yoga or kick-boxing class if your weight is over 300 pounds? Are the requirements for participation in a sport so steeply insurmountable before beginning that you must get in shape just to exercise? Make sure your attitude and aptitude match with what you wish to "enjoy" on an ongoing basis.

In regard to training requirements, let's look at America's pastime. No, not NASCAR! Baseball is a sport requiring sudden bursts of speed after periods of inactivity. Explosiveness is required for batting, fielding, stealing bases and sprinting to first. Any sports which require bat or club swings are best utilized when power production equals shot control, which requires core, lower back, shoulder, forearm, rhomboid and serratus incorporation. The gluteus, hamstrings, inner knee, erector spinea, obliques and lower latissumus are all involved in the simple motion of swinging a bat.

Quick, solid hitting requires flexibility, reflexes, timing and hand-eye coordination. Great spine flexibility is also a must; so these many varied components make up the necessary training to just hit the ball, not accounting for the hand-eye timing and concentration necessary, or the variable dynamics of how the ball is thrown.

The pitcher and catcher do most of the throwing for the duration of the game, so they must be flexible, strong and possess stamina. Short distances of lateral, forward, backward 10-yard sprints, and explosive step-and-sprint movements are executed regularly. Most infield positions work within 4 square yard spaces. The training must mimic the quick, strong leverages and torques required for baseball. Trunk training – front and back - because of left to right to left rotational moves is imperative. These are just the requirements for the simple sport of baseball.

Hockey and soccer are constant motion sports; football, volleyball, golf, and others are stop and go. Sports such as track's field events require a combination unlike other sports, of speed, explosiveness, and/or throwing objects or leaping vertically or horizontally in synchronously-timed bursts of precision.

Basketball covers much ground, with a combination of jumping, turning, sprinting, directional changes, strength, stamina and finesse. Explosiveness is required both vertically and horizontally. Basketball is more of a vertical sport, whereas hockey is more horizontal. So training for basketball should involve leaving the ground, landing, and moving quickly in another direction; while for hockey, short sprints involving many directional changes are the most beneficial.

Know what your sport requires. Learn what foods best supply the fuel necessary for your endeavors. Use the equipment that's required for your safety and assure that it fits correctly and guards properly. Examine all the requirements your sport enlists, and, like your training, incorporate as many facets as possible into practice and play.

Be aware of the requirements of certain sports, of proper shoes, helmets or padding. Having an understanding of basic requirements for your particular sport – basic, just what it takes to get involved – raises your overall awareness of how much more you can learn to incorporate into your preparations for safe, optimal participation.

T *IME*

Time has as many factors as there are minutes in an hour. You must consider how long of a time you spend on the field, how active those minutes are, and what is required for the duration of the contest.

A 3-minute round to a boxer is not the same as three minutes on the football field; it's much time to the boxer, and limited to the football player; to a track sprinter, it's many races, to a marathoner, it's a rest stop. It's all relative and relevant to the sport of choice and the types of training involved.

Time is also the consideration for how long a season lasts, for how much preseason training is required, if there is even an off-season and what must be accomplished then. In the off-season, the time to experiment with new techniques, methods of training, equipment, and treatments allow the brain and body the time to adapt to various conditions. The results build new neurological pathways for the stimulation-response system to recognize patterns of movement and to incorporate them into the nervous system. There are also compensations for changes in bodymass, balance, injuries and age that arise year to year. Simple recuperative downtime must be built into the training schedule. To keep the body and muscles actively surprised and stimulated to respond explosively, training must run in cycles to give the body the ability to adapt through a series of higher stresses toward the designated event or season. The simplest, best way to plot time is with the Timeline.

Time is equal for everyone. If you choose to converse or cavort through your training, then it is ill-spent. If it's utilized to it's fullest, than you've done all you can to get the most out of your time allotment. And your body and performances will respond in kind with superior delivery day after day as only the elite athlete experiences. You do not have to fill every waking hour in the pursuit of your sport. That's unbalanced and unhealthy. But designating time and then honoring it according to the blocks you've plotted is proactive and productive.

S *TRENGTH*

A marathon runner needs strong legs and strong lungs, but in addition, also good core stability, lower back strength, shoulder strength and mental endurance. To just run without conditioning the weaker links will assure injuries and weaknesses down the road. Many runners, sprinters or marathoners, do not realize how important an adequate bench press is for improving the upper body strength required for explosive and prolonged endurance.

You must determine whether you're training for SIZE, STAMINA, SPEED or all three. Is it advantageous to have bulk for your sport? Or is it more important to keep up a high level of energy output for an extended time period? Do you sprint in short bursts while using your upper body often, or does the sport call for explosive action followed by a slower paced interval?

Is strength required for extended, sustained periods as in football or basketball? Or does it serve explosively as in wrestling or boxing,? Is speed a quick trigger, or a rolling buildup of power production, as in a marathon or the steady pacing of swimming? Is proprioception the most important capability for your body as in skiing or gymnastics; or is stable solidity most necessary as with a wrestler or weightlifter?

In baseball, maximum deltoid effort is 110 °, which means the athlete must do high pulls, upright rows, incline bench presses, and military presses in a combination of both pushing and pulling exercises. Shoulder stability and mobility depend upon trapezius and serratus muscles. There is also a direct correlation between body mass and batting power. So getting body mass up while keeping body fat down is crucial.

The components of every sport are so varied and so numerous that to just train everything is as counterproductive as training what you "think" you use in each sport. Training the crucial aspects first, then the general, then any supplementary bodyparts, is the only feasible way to attain a well-rounded regimen which encompasses the training necessary to your sport.

The means of acquiring and maintaining body strength are not some big secret that cannot be tapped. Gaining strength is possible for the 17 or the 70 year old. The only secrets to strength training for specific sports are angles, hand positions, rep schemes and varying loads, with a good knowledge of exercise order. You can be too strong for a sport with inappropriate training. You can be strongly superior in certain lifts and overly weak in critical areas. The more you really think of what your sport requires and how your strength is utilized are the keys to making the most of both.

SPORTS ARE EVERYWHERE

Get out of the "safe zones" of training. Try new exercises, sports, activities. They need not be "extreme sports." Croquet requires skill, strategy, patience and a level of competence, it's competitive but also relaxing and fun. Feel the weight of your body shift, your balance, your timing, in something as mundane as bowling, as frivolous as badminton, as passive as bicycling. Train away from your strengths. Train your weaknesses. Strive for as few weaknesses as possible, rather than growing one "great" strength.

Within a weightlifting exercise, explode in a hard contraction after a slow, steady, full extension of movement. Strength is the basis for power and endurance. Use as many muscles in training as are used in the event, including mental. Most of all, examine the sports you participate in or would like to compete, with critical attention to how the body moves, what the motions are, how much strength is required and the space your position occupies. Then visualize yourself in that position and watch how quickly your body adapts in reaction to the plans set by imagination. Competition, no matter how many players are on the field, comes down to one person who ultimately wants to win, you.

There is beauty in the physical plane. Through our physical nature we transcend earth and achieve the spiritual. All athletes in all sports experience it at some time in their lives. The best achieve it most often. Breaking tackles or cracking home runs, slam dunking, spiking, pinning, acing, slamming, scoring, outracing, hanging ten – everyone has had this feeling, this transcendence. An undisturbed, focused concentration, devoted to the higher development of the physical body, should be no more or less intense than attempting to elevate the spiritual. When this attention is directed toward a particular sport, the results are often higher than original expectations.

"To accomplish great things, we must not only act, but also dream; not only plan, but also believe."
- Anatole Franc

10

<u>SYSTEM</u>

"Whosoever Asserts Himself

Has Will Power

Whosoever Is Self-Sufficient Is Rich."

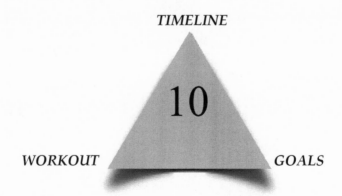

TIMELINE

10

WORKOUT   GOALS

THE SYSTEM

A system is a set of components to draw from and adapt as a way of accomplishing measurable goals through proven means to reach an expected outcome.

To "assert" yourself is to go to the field or the gym alone, and perform your workout, without worrying how much anyone sees you sweat or hears you scream. You build "will power" by going against it when you don't feel like training, and train anyway. By "asserting" yourself time and time again, facing the same challenges in the discipline you've chosen, your "will" soon takes that insurmountable weight, that monotonous run, that impossible pose, and conquers it through perseverance. As you get stronger, so too does your will and as your will gets stronger, so too do you.

To grow "rich" in self-sufficiency is to face the many trials of training and continuously prove to your mind that "you can, you can, you can," erasing all doubts with results. To be "self-sufficient" is to know how to make up a workout with little or no equipment, but still make the exercise challenging. By exhibiting "will power" and becoming "self-sufficient" you develop a system, a workout repertoire, a health regimen, and the ways and means for you to improve your game and your life.

A system gives you guidelines to follow, to check and balance your training on a daily, weekly, monthly and yearly basis. But it is not set in stone. Adaptation must be allowed to compensate for changes that occur along the way.

You use a system for eating, for training, for rest. You need to follow some type of guidelines for a certain period of time, then keep what works and discard what doesn't. The system is simply your way of gathering results to make your training, body, life and sport measurably better. The system always works toward improvement, despite having to break things down to get to there.

Following a system means facing the day with the knowledge that you will do something to work on your fitness on that day, and that what you set yourself up to accomplish will be done. Day 2 builds on day 1. You find you did too much or not enough, and then find the balance of what can be done on the next workout. When you go back the next week, increase the duration or the intensity. Duration will increase stamina and endurance, while intensity will increase size, shape and speed. Both duration and intensity are necessary to get the most out of your workouts, but must be done with balance.

THE TIMELINE

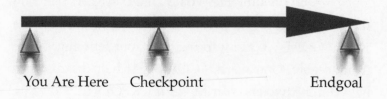

You Are Here   Checkpoint   Endgoal

POSITIVE HABITS/GOALS

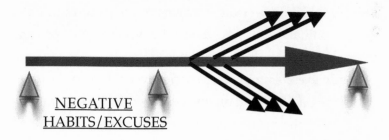

NEGATIVE
HABITS/EXCUSES

- Positive habits get you to where you desire to be;
- Negative habits and excuses take you away from your goals, and your destination.

THE TIMELINE SYSTEM

Draw a timeline. Write, "YOU ARE HERE", on the far left end of it. On the right side of the timeline write, "GOAL". Write it in big, standout lettering. Make it noticeable. One word, "GOAL". At half the distance between the two ends write, "CHECKPOINT".

Record your current statistics at the left end under "YOU ARE HERE;" what is your current weight, strength, weakness, limitation and whatever else you feel will nail down exactly where you stand on this date, your initial starting date. If you're 40 pounds overweight, admit it; inflexible, state it; or if you are already exercising once or twice a week, record the good with the bad. Make it an absolutely critical assessment.

At the checkpoint, record, right now, how much you feel you can honestly move toward your goal in that allotted time. Unrealistic goals don't happen. Make it a practical, reasonable, tangent idea or vision you can hold on to and reach. If that checkpoint goal is possible, than the end goal becomes even more possible.

The "End Goal" is the one you can exaggerate because what often happens is you surpass it prior to the actual date. If you work with conviction and perseverance toward that end goal, 10 out of 11 times, you reach it. All you need to add is your willingness through "self-sufficient willpower." Assert your will to be better and you will be better.

THE WORKOUT SYSTEM

Do 2 sets of 11 repetitions of multiple joint warm ups such as Dips for chest, Lunges for legs and Pull Ups for back. Then, pick a major exercise from each body part section. Choose a multiple-joint movement, such as the Bench Press for chest; the Squat for legs or Barbell Rows for back.

4 sets of 11 repetitions to build, with a compound, multiple joint movement

Perform 4 x 11 reps of this first compound movement, as heavy as possible with strict form. Form shapes the muscle, not the weight. Do the first exercise with a weight heavy enough to challenge yourself for 11 repetitions. If you make 11 reps, add weight the second set, subtract weight if you don't. If you make it to 11 reps again on the second set, add a little more weight for the third and fourth sets, again, only if perfect form and control are held throughout the repetitions. Each week, the starting set weight can be increased as well as each subsequent set. This means progress.

When you get sloppy, stop, drop weight, or rest for 20 seconds and then complete the set. Always get all the repetitions regardless of how much weight you must drop to get there. This is a way of telling your muscles you are not giving in or quitting. Persevere and the next time you'll take less stops to get to 11. You should push to finish but don't let the movement get sloppy or ruin good, strict form. Soon, there will be no stops and you'll be adding weight. You'll know then the System is working.

4 sets for the same bodypart from another angle

Now choose a second exercise that incorporates the same body part, but from a different angle; Incline or Decline Bench Press for chest; Leg Press or Lunges for legs; Seated Pulley Rows or Pull Downs for back. This is your second movement from a different angle for 4 x 11 repetitions. Use the same guidelines to add weight each set.

3 sets of a specific movement to shape and refine with added concentration

The third movement will be more specific to the particular bodypart you're working. Specific movements target the one muscle group and usually involve single-joint exercises, isolating the muscle so that only that muscle is doing the work. Dumbbell Flies or Cable Crossovers for chest, with arms in a slightly bent but locked in position so the pectorals are engaged in the movement exclusively; Leg Curls or Extensions for legs, where the quadriceps and hamstrings do the majority of the work; and Single Arm Dumbbell Rows, as an example, though working any part of the back usually requires other joint involvement due to the large range of motion necessary for proper back training.

THE GOAL SYSTEM

When beginning a strength training program, the first goals usually involve disciplining your body to go to the gym a certain number of days in a row and doing certain required movements a certain number of times. Once you become familiar with the workout regimens, you start adding weight or repetition goals, performance goals, timed goals, nutrition goals and aesthetic goals.

The experience of feeling the changes your body is going through accelerate the type and number of possibilities, hence goals, you set for yourself. Momentum creates outcomes often over and above the original plans and motivation comes easier when visible results are confirmed and felt through feedback by yourself and others who notice the transformations taking place. The mind feeds on positive reinforcement, enabling the body to transcend any limiting ideals that may stand in the way. You can pat or smack a dog. He'll stretch to receive one thing while cowering from the other.

We are the same animals when noticing if anyone notices, or shirking away when wishing to be avoided or invisible. Please yourself first, then notice the pleasant effect it has on others.

The rewards found in goal achievement should first and foremost be for the self-development and preservation of you and your body toward your goal or sport. The recognition of others is secondary and should never be the means for what we set out to achieve, doing things to spite or disprove an opinion not of our own. Passion and energy drive the athlete, while anger and envy are the brakes that literally break the athlete's drive. Fire is beneficial only when it is controlled, directed and properly utilized. With goals, the metaphoric fire burns clean and steadily, consuming only what it needs rather than everything in its path, which ultimately leads to distinction instead of destruction

S.Y.S.T.E.M.

S *TRATEGY* –A realistic, step-by-step plan for a certain achievement.

Y *EARLY* – Working toward the big picture while achieving little victories

S *YNERGY* – Makes all aspects of your workouts work in your favor, no weak links.

T *RIAL* – Strength, Speed, Flexibility and Concentration training are essential.

E *LEMENTS* – What will it take in effort, time, equipment and instruction?

M *OTIVATION* – Set your goals, see the good, and work in forward, positive actions.

S *TRATEGY*

One of the best things to do for effective workouts is to plan them in advance. Once you work with them for a few weeks, and fall into the routine of the order of movements with strict specifics to their execution, you can make nearly any half hour in any gym productive. When you work in your regular gym, get into the habit of using the same stations in the same order, a number of times in a row. When it feels stale and non-productive, add one or two different movements at a time until you've replaced all the old movements with new ones. You can also reverse the exercise order for variety.

Having a plan ensures you will accomplish x amount in y time. The variable will be the intensity you bring to it. The strategy for all these types of training should be kept simple and structured. This assures that they're measurable, balanced, thorough and achievable.

You should perform your hardest work, the furthest from your season. As you get closer to it, your momentum and motivation will be high and that much easier to get through the finer details that make no sense to concentrate on nine months out. Doing the hardest first also builds character and discipline that carries you through the year. If your goal is to simply be in the best swimsuit shape by June, your most challenging workouts have to happen in January and February, or ultimately, the previous October. This mentality applies to whatever your Endgoal will be.

Your strategy should involve learning as much as you need to learn, acquiring as many tools as necessary to add value to the training, and eliminating as many weaknesses as possible, whether physical, mental or spiritual.

Be open to disciplines like yoga, Pilates, meditation, visualization, stretching, praying, observing and the smorgasbord of activities that aren't your particular sport.

The best things often come effortlessly, or seem to be effortless. This happens when efficiency of motion, range of motion, and explosive or directional motions are rote. The practice comes in play, and consistently superior play comes in practice.

Y *EARLY*

A yearly plan can be as simple as, "being in better shape than last year," or, as tough as "cutting minutes off next spring's marathon." A yearly focus is important to keep you centered and on track for whatever your athletic endeavor may be. If you wish to improve your golf handicap, do something you hadn't tried before, like Pilates or yoga for better balance and flexibility, or some form of meditation to sharpen concentration skills. Weight training and extra cardiovascular training are measurable ways to improve your function in sports, so always strive to try new equipment, exercises or disciplines.

All the aspects within a system of training for any sport should be done in 4, 4 and 3 month segments, with 1 complete month of rest, review and recharging. Many things can be done year round, but priorities should vary throughout each year and season. If you're training for no sport in particular, then your yearly season is "life". What do you wish to work on to improve this year? Every single one of us has room for improvement. Everyone!

If you can feasibly see into the next year, it enables you to sustain a vigilant pace for the season and training you're currently involved in. Yearly goals give you breathing room as you see that all changes need not be hurried through; but with consistent, dedicated effort, are sure to come about. Focusing on the year also helps to realize when things aren't coming as quickly as anticipated, and that more work is necessary to achieve the stated goal.

Breaking commitments into 3 or 4 month segments throughout a year allows compensation for injuries, setbacks, personal issues, and reevaluations to be methodically approached and the training to stay on course. There are many ways to break a year down, but by keeping the long term in mind while accomplishing little victories keeps the motivation high and the results recognizable.

S YNERGY

Synergy means to take the physical aspect of strength training and combine it with the flexibility training in a stretching, yoga or Pilates program. The combined attention of these two components makes each of them stronger than individually standing alone. Add the applied efforts of eating correctly and sleeping completely and rather than one pointed effort in a particular discipline, you're adding all these aspects together to multiply the training affects of each other in a synergistic, compounding benefit which brings all three aspects as well as the total system to work better.

Make all aspects of your workouts work in your favor, allow no weak links. Synergy is a blend of all things working seamlessly without interference from interruption, distraction, or lack of vision. Synergy is rare and should be appreciated. It is seldom and far between. But when practice and rehearsal take precedence, the result is often equal to the work put in and more often surpassed.

Synergy is to bring all these facets together – training, nutrition, practice, and rest. By finding the optimum exercises for your body type and sport, you'll continually move in a positive direction each season. When you find the right foods to eat to keep you both satisfied and lean, and their proper proportions, you'll experience the best health you could ever treat your body to. By knowing your body enough to know when to push it and when to rest, you'll find balance, strength, clarity and confidence. In finding synergy, the practice takes over and becomes almost automatic, effortless and sometimes, enjoyable!

T *RIAL*

This is the one definitive aspect in the System that separates every athlete from each other, Trial. Figure out what works for your body, your lifestyle, your timeline, your abilities, your tastes, your budget, your aptitude, your environment, your head and your heart. There is no one form of exercise or apparatus or movement or food which is universally accepted and embraced, no secret pills, diets, medallions or chants that will give you what you're searching for in physicality until you try a number of avenues and disciplines and settle on a System of health and fitness that is unique to your desires. Bodybuilders have known this throughout the ages and are responsible for so much of the experimenting in movements and eating habits that have given the general public the most insight into harnessing superior performance from their bodies and creating the aesthetic appeal so many common people strive to achieve. Try many things, wholeheartedly, systematically and attentively.

Trial in regard to the system also has to do with evaluating techniques on a regular basis, as a way to check in to test if the desired benefits are coming. With weight-lifting movements, you must periodically test your strength in maximum lifts to qualify if the techniques are garnering more strength in specific lifts from 3 months prior. Endurance, flexibility or whatever the particular movement is utilized to achieve, must be tried at given intervals in the system training cycle to ensure the correct approach is performed.

Trial is a check and balance system that makes the rest of the training accountable to the goals, cycles, season, and sports you are training toward. You do not begin running 20 miles a day one month before a marathon to get in shape for it, you plot out your timeline, begin with short runs and strength workouts to alleviate any weak links and as your body responds to the effects of each training regimen, you alter, adapt and eliminate accordingly. By trial we alleviate errors.

E *LEMENTS*

The Elements represent the basic ingredients you will need to properly execute your workouts and a fitness lifestyle. Be certain that you set your schedule to accommodate your goals for the week. Map your plan out, the order of exercises, the types of weights you'll attempt, the new movements you will try and the times spent in each discipline each week. A schedule is just as much an element as having a barbell.

Be certain to have a partner, trainer or spotter available on heavy lifting days; a facility where proper stretching can be done and apparatus for your flexibility training; a field or court to do plyometrics and sprint training; a market that offers fresh fruits, meats, vegetables and nuts for proper nourishment and a place for vitamin supplements that has a knowledgeable staff and reasonably priced products. These elements are all part of your system, which will ensure you move through your physical life as smoothly as any other aspect of it.

The system elements are comprised of everything from your game plan to the post-workout meal you'll consume. Certain cycles require certain supplements for better performance and the availability and timely consumption of things like protein, creatine, amino acids and multi-vitamins are each elements which comprise the make-up of a successful training cycle.

Everything involved in your sport of choice should be inspected regularly for breaks or potentially dangerous flaws that may need tuning up, replacement or binding. Your physical body should not have any weak links, so why would your equipment. It is up to you to make certain every element contributes to your welfare instead of detracting or limiting it in any way. The elements in your system are all the things necessary to keep your peace of mind as well as optimum performance.

M OTIVATION

This is something that is a constant. There is no question if this is essential or not. If it is not there, neither are you. Motivation not only takes you from here to the goal line, it gets you from A to Z and anywhere in between. Being motivated should not be confused with "going through the motions." Motivation is a must, concentration is a must. Surgeons and musicians don't just "go through the motions" even though their occupations require repetitive tasks.

If it takes employing someone else to motivate you, spend the money. If that is what requires you to get to your workout, find someone to help you show up, guide you, encourage, account for and motivate you. But ultimately you must motivate yourself to improve your health, because if a negative diagnosis was the alternative offering, you would get motivated very fast to get better! You would do whatever it takes by any means necessary and find time as well as the best help available.

In your wake you will create a following, sweeping loved ones along to share in this noticeably better feeling. When people see you improving, they will ask what you are doing. Guaranteed. You will motivate in just doing.

Motivation grows just like the rest of a workout and your body, in increments. Your motivation waxes and wanes, it expands or compresses. As long as it is always present, as long as you are consistently making it to the gym, motivation will be there too. If you can reduce your weight and increase your strength with the dogged determination that you put into getting out of shape, consistently doing "something" instead of consistently doing "nothing," motivation will radiate from you with a positive wealthiness that others will try to get from you. You may as well share your motivation. It only helps yours grow.

THOUGHT, WORD & DEED

THOUGHT, WORD & DEED are the summary for SYSTEM. If you feel uncomfortable in your body, either by pain, performance or ability, you must draw your thoughts to improvement. Once it's thought out, you write a plan with goals or find a workout you'd like to follow. You can add strength and stability to your torso, add power to your swing, or speed to your movement. But you must lay out a plan to follow and then follow through, by showing up, one day, ready to exercise. The showing up, the attempt, by sheer diligence and perseverance is the deed that proves to your mind and outline that you're capable of change and improvement.

The more you begin THINKING of how you'd like to change your body, the better the PLAN you create to move toward your goals. The clearer the plan and vision the more effective each workout becomes. The more focused and specific the exercises, the sooner you reach your physical goals. The results, in turn, lead you back to thinking MORE about your workouts, body, and diet; leading to more plans, more workouts, more results. Paying attention is what it's all about. The less you care about your body and your health, the more it goes away – literally and figuratively. The closer the attention, the better, faster and more continuous the development. Maintenance becomes The Way. You develop a Strategy for Yearly improvement. You incorporate Synergy through Trial of all the Elements, bringing them together with consistent Motivation toward ultimate yet evolving goals. You have in place, a SYSTEM. A Simple, Structured Training system. SST!

"When I say always, I mean forever, and that's a mighty long time..." - Prince

11

<u>FOREVER</u>

"Whosoever Does Not Lose His Place

Has Duration.

Whosoever Does Not Perish In Death

Lives.

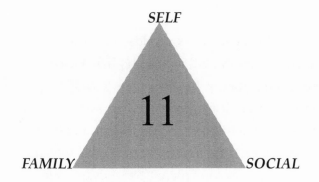

FOREVERLAND

You will never "lose your place" as long as you keep adapting, experimenting, believing, trying and applying. By having an open mind and great faith, you will endure. We need to be fully engaged in the welfare of the body we're given to fulfill our space in life. Doctors, therapists, Holistic practitioners, trainers and "club pros" can educate, instruct, manipulate and advise, but it is up to each of us individually to create ideal states and environments for our bodies to endure. By defining our influences we retain our own longevity.

Did you ever wonder why teachers don't seem to age? Because they continually embrace changes and new ways of looking at old things. They never "lose their place" because their set point continually adapts. Their "place" is a connected progression of points along a timeline and their lives are "youth-filled. " They have "duration."

DO NOT LOSE YOUR PLACE

"Whosoever does not lose his place" is the man or woman standing tall in their bodies. When we choose responsibility for our health, we seek knowledge of how to best maintain it on each level. To keep our "place" is to admit responsibility for the honor to be as healthy and active participants as possible in this life we're granted. We "lose our place" by giving power to those ready to tell us what we wish to hear and take money for all the things we don't need, the quick fixes and band aids that mask healing. We relinquish our own power over duration. "Duration" means going the distance, but it also means having the strength in reserve all along the way for performance, healing and sharing. We will last when we put ourselves first, and in so doing, "live."

"Whosoever does not perish in death lives." Do you know anyone who has died in mind, body or spirit before leaving earth? Those who have lost their will, who have given in to disease and inactivity and therefore, "perished" by choosing not to live fully?

To "not perish in death" means to live in every moment of every day, even if it's spent reading a book under a tree. Refuse to buy in to disease, thinking science can "fix" you. Medicine should be the last refuge, not the first. Diet pills, invasive surgeries, and the "healthful" fixes that are performed with you in a chair or on a gurney are not really doing anyone any good except the person performing the "fix." You stay youthful by doing youth filled activities and practices. A baby eats, sleeps, plays, bends and eliminates instinctively when it needs to. At what point did we lose that common sense?

Remember to balance the Family, Social and Self aspects of living by participating in each sector. Your influence toward health can reach others in the oddest ways and places. Family activities can involve anything from biking to cooking healthy meals. Your social life can contain events and activities that enhance your memories rather than rot them away! The things you do for your self can be the reflection that others need to see in themselves; and therefore the mind, body and even soul will grow in influence, importance and "duration" and will not "perish in death," but live in posterity as those examples tumble down generations.

FOR EVER

The morning light was enough to determine the outside temperature, dictating what clothes we'd wear, which were usually the same clothes as yesterday, stacked in a heap on the floor. We'd bound to breakfast, happy, well-rested. We'd had dreams to recall and cereal, toast and orange juice before we could leave. We'd care about how the day was headed, often from plans made with three friends the day before. If nothing panned out, we still chose activity over anything sedentary. Driving in a car for any period was devastating. Going shopping, excruciating. Inventing games was a pastime, and daydreaming, a prerequisite to play.

When we ran it was effortless, it was fast, it was often, and it was painless. We ran every day and we ran everywhere. We ran forever. Or rode. Bikes were just an extension of our arms and legs. We biked for miles and in sprints between each other's homes, going extra fast when dinner was on the table. We ate regularly scheduled meals and ate all that was in front of us, down to the last nasty lima bean.

At 11, we didn't know yet what we couldn't do, so we tried most everything. Fearlessly. Superman and Spiderman, Wonder Woman and Tarzan were our heroes. We viewed things from a perspective higher than life because we were on top and above it. Our heroes were athletes and icons who never did wrong. We all aspired to be someone great.

Everyone knew where each friend was on any given day. Play was embraced as much as eating or sleeping. Dinner was that inconvenience between innings. And when we played good, that play looped over and over in our consciousness until the next great memory came along to replace it. The more we played, the better we slept, and the better we slept, the brighter each day looked.

As men and women we tend to recall our years as boys and girls. We remember moments and liken them to a feeling we'd experienced as children or teens, somewhere on a playing field. The way we ran, the way we felt, the way we moved so free and easy, was taken for granted. We played with no end in sight. And we never got tired!

The benefits gained from sports stay with us for many years. The memories and visualizations reoccur in boardrooms, when managing projects, initiating ideas, creating metaphors for superiors to believe in, or recollecting victories, and reminiscing with teammates who've now become neighbors and friends and coaches and partners.

As grown ups we try to pretend there's no time for recreation, or we go to extremes when we find a space of time only to end up sore and aching for weeks instead of invigorated because we'd overdone it or done it wrong.

Young men and women should learn proper body maintenance regardless if they're athletes or not, as long as we live in a gravity-based world. When future generations live in space or spend extended times there, you can be sure that they're doing weight training here on earth. It will be and should be a way of life for everyone, now. Proper instruction at an early age contributes to a person's self esteem, medical health, confidence, security, safety and their chances of participating at team sports by constantly proving what they can do, and ingraining it in themselves as part of their makeup. When you show someone how to pick themselves up off the floor, they'll be down there less often.

By learning basic exercises for the core and the body parts, lifelong health, vitality, energy, flexibility and the pursuit of many varied adventures and challenges will ensure fulfillment on many levels that technology cannot. Human performance is absolutely remarkable. The feats that still astonish are physical. Men, women and children of every culture indulge in sport at some time in their lives. We even realize how important and beneficial it is for the handicapped to compete in a safe and natural way. Training can be done in a 4 x 4 bedroom or a 4400 foot mountain meadow. It can be done in seriously intent concentration or unbridled, abandoning joy. The benefits are endless.

F. O. R .E .V .E .R.

F *LOW* – body and lifestyle together to the end.

O *WNERSHIP* - Pride and care of possessions.

R *EWARD* - Everything you do to improve your mind and body rewards you.

E *NHANCEMENT* – The more areas you focus on positively, the less negatives you have.

V ALUE - Exercise and activity are usually free, unlike hospital visits!

E *SCAPE* - Release the mind and body to new freedoms and heights.

R *EMEMBER* – The good through accomplishments, the bad in limitations.

F *LOW*

Flow happens when the automatic response of an event is accepted and responded to by the body in an unthinking yet deeply intuitive way. It's when we catch something thrown to us without looking, by just reacting. It's like coloring with a child without any expectation or constraint, yet often a pleasing result occurs from the mindless attention given to filling in the blanks. Flow is the Zen-like occurrence where all motion seems to go around you, while still encompassing and transporting without force.

Nature has patterns that have always been and always will be. Water moves. Wind moves. Land moves. Fire moves. Fire isn't just the fever, it's the eternal pilot light that burns until we pass from this existence; but still, our energy lives on. We are all of these things too. Thoughts of us, things we've left, experienced with others, written – all flow long after we're gone.

Flow is a part of life. You must just be more aware of its presence and it will take you anywhere you wish to go. If you fight it, try to force it or direct it, you will be met with greater opposition than you can ever handle. Nature will win. You will break down. Learn flow by practicing simple daily regimens, by making healthful, intelligent choices and by choosing movement over stagnation. Be loose. Flow.

O *WNERSHIP*

What you have is what you get. But the body you were born with is not the body you carry to the grave. If you are proud of it, take good care of it, maintain it regularly, give it good fuel and supply adequate rest, you will proudly keep it polished and show it off. If you neglect it, starve it, overindulge it or ignore it, these things will all show and the resulting weaknesses will manifest as flaws in physique, physicality and health. You'll attract disease, harbor injuries and lean on what's lacking rather than concentrate on strengths.

How you choose to own your body is reflected in how you would own any other object. If you respect yourself and your health, you'll be rewarded with the same in equal measure. If you abuse it and take it for granted, your rewards will be a bruised lifestyle full of setbacks and restrictions, pain and ugly occurrences that in the end will deform your body and wreck your spirit. Your body will be the "beater" on the highway of life.

You not only own the physical aspect of your life, you own the thoughts and the results of that thinking too. If you continually think you "never can or never will", you won't! You'll prove yourself right. But even in trying, even in failed attempts, with an attitude that we are indeed working toward improvement, we grow in positive directions. By constantly "owning" our thoughts, feelings and actions, we claim what's possible. And when we see what's possible, we expand our beliefs, experiences, attempts and accomplishments, in every endeavor. We only fail when we give up. Your body, mind and spirit are the only things you truly own in this lifetime. All else comes and goes. Take care of it, and own all its benefits.

R EWARD

When you learn something new and it enthuses you, you desire to share it and its benefits. You are rewarded with the grace to give. You share healthy foods and positive activities. You are interested in the welfare of, and helpful toward the ones you love dearest, guiding but not directing, informing but not berating. You find an interest in gaining knowledge about yourself and the things that are considered obstacles in daily life. These are all rewards. The value you place in self-preservation and maintenance is the reward you will cherish for a lifetime.

Each sore muscle, each bead of sweat, each strained breath to stride another step, is a reward. The pain is released as pleasure immediately on completion. Anyone who thinks this self-inflicted beating isn't worth the reward should ask someone who cannot perform it; ask a quadriplegic or the bed-bound obese to trade places. Those who come from those depths and succeed are the true heroes in our culture, the real icons to be revered. The reward is in doing, and as long as you can, do. Because once you absolutely cannot, it's an entirely different story.

An hour of exercise gives back days of stress reduction, months to your life, and a commitment, focus and dedication almost as strong as any human bond. You are consistently rewarded with the benefits of spending time in the gym or on the field. The more you learn about exercise and the more you share it, the more you get back. The more you practice it, the easier it gets and the rewards continue expanding.

E NHANCEMENT

People must learn to embrace the concept of exercise as a good thing, not just a necessary thing. You feel good when you're done, you feel as if you've accomplished something you started out not wanting to attempt. Exercise keeps you in touch with your body. Your body is your vehicle, it's not just a dwelling. It needs care, maintenance, and upkeep. It needs to be as flexible and fluid as it needs to be solid. The mind needs to be challenged, the lungs need aeration, and the joints need pliability and resilience. The more completely one learns to exercise, the more completely they will rest to recuperate. It's a simple cycle. The more attention paid is the more attention given. If it's done in a positive, optimistic, rewarding fashion, the actions are preventative of sickness and disease. If it's done regretfully, you are looking for things to go wrong. You find blame, aches and excuses to not learn more about your pursuits, your physique and your future.

Embrace the goodness found in exercise. Exercise your mind, body and spirit. Each step toward health is two steps away from sickness. Momentum carries you forward. Resistance pulls you back. Even attempting to exercise benefits the body, even if you fail the endeavor. Failure means successfully finding what works and what doesn't. Every activity either enhances or degrades your life. Choose only those that enhance the body, mind and spirit to stay on the high roads of living.

Enhance the experience of every workout by watching how others do the same movements, by continually testing yourself rather than going through the motions, by trying new aspects and regimens, by reading to grow in the knowledge of what the body is doing in particular planes of motion and to keep abreast of new findings to benefit your sport or lifestyle. When you enhance the workout experience through an open-minded approach, you automatically open new avenues which weren't previously available to your body.

V ALUE

There is no true amount that can be attributed to Value. If exercise extends your life for 11 extra years, how valuable is that? What will you see and what would you miss? To be able to move freely, without restriction, is as valuable at 77 as being able to do a cartwheel at 11. Friends are immobile and you can climb 6 flights of stairs without an extra breath; how valuable is that? How valuable are a few extra breaths during sex?

Value comes in volumes. When you begin to value the interest in your body that exercise affords, you begin to see that, not only is physical change possible, but also changes in your thinking about capabilities toward any other goals. All is possible.

Of all possessions, health is the one you can most control. When your health is out of control, it is only your fault. When it is at its best, placed as your highest value, it is your blessing, and the residual effects to those around you are contagious.

Exercise improves everything. It adds internal, structural, organ and emotional health benefits. It's a stress reliever, hormone releaser, endurance builder, V02-Max increaser, immunity booster, sex drive enhancer; esteem, confidence, will, goal setting, and discipline builder. You look better, stand taller, eat better, think more clearly, stay focused for longer periods, have better stamina, better sex and create stronger offspring through action and example. And, more clothes fit, better!

Value not only the activities found in fitness, but the time allowed to pursue them. If you are only given an hour every other day, utilize it, look forward to it, plan it, pursue it and therefore get the most value from it. The droning lumps taking up space across gym floors everywhere are not appreciative of the value workout time affords. The busy housewife, the overworked laborer, the driven businessman and woman, still find one minuscule increment of time to fit in a workout and make the most of it. So should you, for those are the real "golden moments."

E SCAPE

Do not think of exercise as running away from something. Think of it as running TOWARD something. When you run to health, you enlist all your senses to the cause of becoming something you currently are not. You always strive to change for the better. You NEVER work to change for the worse. Giving in is effortless. Giving more is work. Strange how we always seem to give more when we reach the most. Exercise grounds you as equally as it elevates you.

When you pay attention and internalize the movement, you progress at a pace 11 times that of the average trainee. When you go through the motions and take up nothing more than floor space, you get results slightly more than those who choose not to come. You must value the time you have to work on yourself as sacred, and you must religiously dictate to your mind what you wish it to accomplish. You will see the changes and more if you believe them as you commit them to your goals. Be realistic but not simplistic. Any single thing you set out for your body to accomplish can be attained, at any age. Believe that sincerely. You'll reach something close enough resembling your goal to encourage you to continue toward excellence. Refined focus comes in eternally reaching.

Time spent on yourself is a chance to escape the demands of the day and give you something to look forward to on a regular basis. Your body thrives on the regularity that exercise induces, the hormones it releases, the blood flow, oxygen flow, focus and satisfaction it allows by just getting away from the extraneous noise and getting into the moments of concentrated effort required to train properly. Escape into your life, rather than from it, and reclaim it as your own through exercise, health and fitness.

R EMEMBER

Let the low points be a catalyst for inspiration as well as the high points. It's easy to recall your best game, the magic moments, the highlights of your youth; but also remember the periods when you were too fat or too slow or injured, and remember especially how you got in those conditions – by not exercising, by not working on your game, by being lazy or neglectful or less thorough in your attention to preparation.

Those are the moments to remember, so you'll never be that fat kid again, the last one picked in pick up games, the one who usually sat the bench. Let those times remind you that the past does not equal the future. You can be stronger, more agile, more flexible, leaner, lighter, quicker, more durable, focused, and desirable. Think of a car left in a garage for many years, the tires are flattened on one side, the structure squeaks, rattles and moans from non-use, from inactivity. So too does the sedentary body.

By starting slow, maintaining control, and watching the vital signs, you pick up speed and with speed, momentum. If you throw your body haphazardly at life, at your game, you're destined to crash sooner or later. If you check and balance, expand and contract, risk and assess, learn and grow, you will go further, at faster speeds with safer results.

Exercise must be a "forever" proposition. You wouldn't buy a car and stop taking care of it after 2 years. You can't expect high performance out of your body by taking care of it in spurts. Your body works mechanically, parts break down. With intelligent attention, you'll stay away from replacement parts and out of the junkyard. Remember, as long as you eat and sleep in this gravity-based world, you must exercise, in some way, forever.

What "**FOREVER**" means to me

There was a roller blade trail I used to skate on every lunch hour. I was closing in on 40 years old, had my third son, and looked forward to a trip to Scottsdale, Arizona in a few months. I was in the best shape of my life in a life filled with great shape. I had goals, time, determination, perseverance and will. The trail had a few hills, some good straight-aways, smooth pavement and challenging curves.

I had just passed a walking man for the third time. He was probably in his late 60's. Finally, he was able to catch me before I'd passed, with the question, "What are you training for? " He had a smirk on his face, as if he expected some "triathlon" response, like he discovered me, or spied some elite, secret drill since my intensity was so joyfully evident. But I looked back without losing stride and said with a smirk of my own, "Life!"

Printed in Great Britain
by Amazon.co.uk, Ltd.,
Marston Gate.